LIVING WELL

WITH

DIABETES

FOR THE

NEWLY DIAGNOSED

Empowering Yourself for an Awesome and Fulfilling Life on the Journey to Better Health

Catherine CLARKSON

TABLE OF CONTENTS

INTRODUCTION

Welcome to Your New Journey with Diabetes

Welcome, dear reader, to a new chapter in your life. If you're holding this book, you might be grappling with the recent diagnosis of diabetes, and I want you to know that you're not alone. In the pages that follow, we embark on a journey together—a journey of understanding, acceptance, and ultimately, living well with diabetes.

Being diagnosed with diabetes can feel like stepping into an unknown realm, filled with questions, concerns, and perhaps a touch of anxiety. The initial moments of realization can be overwhelming, raising a myriad of emotions. You may wonder, "How will this impact my daily life? What changes do I need to make? Can I still enjoy the things I love?" These questions are not only valid but essential to the process of adapting to this new reality.

So, take a deep breath, and let's navigate this journey together. Diabetes is not a destination; it's a path we walk each day, learning, adjusting, and thriving. The goal of this book is to provide you with the knowledge, tools, and support to live a fulfilling life despite the challenges that diabetes may present.

Understanding Diabetes: Beyond the Diagnosis

Before we delve into the practical aspects of managing diabetes, let's start by understanding what it truly means. Diabetes is not just a medical condition; it's a journey that requires a holistic approach. Whether you're dealing with Type 1 or Type 2 diabetes, the fundamentals remain the same—your body's ability to regulate blood sugar levels is affected.

In the chapters ahead, we'll explore the various types of diabetes, the factors that contribute to its development, and dispel common myths surrounding this condition. Knowledge is a powerful tool, and by understanding diabetes on a deeper level, you'll be better equipped to make informed decisions about your health.

Navigating the Diagnosis: From Shock to Empowerment

The moment you receive a diabetes diagnosis can be a seismic shift in your life. It's okay to feel a mix of emotions—shock, denial, fear, or even anger. Acknowledge these feelings; they are a natural part of the process. In this section, we'll discuss strategies for coping with the initial shock, building a support system around you, and effective communication with healthcare providers.

You are not alone on this journey. Family, friends, and healthcare professionals are here to offer support and guidance. Together, we'll explore ways to transform this initial period of uncertainty into a foundation for empowerment.

Embracing Lifestyle Changes: A New Perspective on Living Well

Diabetes often calls for lifestyle changes, particularly in the realms of diet and physical activity. The key is not to view these changes as restrictions but as opportunities for positive transformation. In the upcoming chapters, we'll delve into the importance of a balanced diet, smart food choices, and incorporating physical activity into your routine.

You don't have to become a fitness guru or a culinary expert overnight. Small, sustainable changes can lead to significant improvements in your overall well-being. This section is not about depriving yourself but about making choices that align with your health goals and contribute to a vibrant, fulfilling life.

Medications and Insulin Management: Navigating Treatment Options

Understanding your treatment options is crucial for effectively managing diabetes. Whether you're exploring oral medications, insulin therapy, or a combination of both, this section provides an in-depth look at the choices available. We'll discuss the types of insulin, methods of administration, and how to manage potential side effects.

Your healthcare team is your ally in finding the right treatment plan for you. By demystifying the world of medications and insulin, we aim to empower you with the knowledge needed to actively participate in decisions about your health.

Monitoring Blood Sugar Levels: Your Health Dashboard

Regular monitoring of blood sugar levels is a cornerstone of diabetes management. In this section, we'll guide you through the process, from selecting a glucose meter to interpreting your readings. Understanding the patterns of your blood sugar levels empowers you to make informed choices about your diet, physical activity, and overall lifestyle.

Setting target ranges, recognizing highs and lows, and adapting your routine accordingly are skills that will become second nature with time. Think of monitoring as your health dashboard, providing real-time insights into how your body responds to different factors.

Preventing Complications: Long-Term Health and Wellness

Diabetes, when managed well, allows for a full and vibrant life. This section focuses on preventing long-term complications by addressing various aspects of your health. We'll delve into cardiovascular health, eye and vision care, kidney health, and the importance of maintaining good foot care.

By understanding the potential complications and taking proactive steps, you'll be better equipped to safeguard your overall well-being. This is not a journey of fear but one of empowerment, where knowledge becomes a shield against potential challenges.

Emotional Well-Being: Nurturing Your Mind and Spirit

Living with diabetes involves more than just managing physical health; it's also about nurturing your emotional well-being. Stress, anxiety, and emotional challenges are natural companions on this journey, but they don't have to define it. In this section, we'll explore strategies for dealing with stress, overcoming emotional challenges, and the importance of seeking professional support when needed.

Your mental and emotional health are integral components of your overall well-being. By addressing these aspects, you'll find greater resilience and a positive outlook on your journey with diabetes.

Living a Full and Active Life: Beyond the Diagnosis

Diabetes doesn't define you; it's just one aspect of your life. This section encourages you to embrace a full and active life by exploring topics such as travel, socializing, dining out, and pursuing hobbies. With the right knowledge and preparation, you can continue to enjoy the activities you love while effectively managing your diabetes.

This is a celebration of life—a reminder that diabetes, though a part of your story, is not the whole story. By living fully, you create a narrative of strength, resilience, and joy.

Conclusion: Your Ongoing Journey of Empowerment

As we conclude this introduction, remember that this book is your companion on a journey of empowerment. Living well with diabetes is not a one-time achievement but an ongoing process of learning, adapting, and thriving. The challenges you face are growth opportunities, and the choices you make today shape the quality of your tomorrow.

You are not defined by your diagnosis; you are defined by your resilience, your choices, and your commitment to living a fulfilling life. Let this book be a guide, a source of inspiration, and a reminder that you have the strength within you to navigate this journey with grace.

Welcome to your new journey with diabetes—a journey of understanding, empowerment, and living well.

CHAPTER 1

Understanding Diabetes: Types, Causes, and Symptoms

Diabetes is a complex and multifaceted condition that affects millions of people worldwide. In this chapter, we will embark on a comprehensive exploration of the various aspects of diabetes, aiming to deepen your understanding of its types, causes, and the common symptoms that serve as crucial indicators of this condition.

Different Types of Diabetes: Overview and Distinctions

Diabetes is not a one-size-fits-all condition; rather, it encompasses a spectrum of types, each with its distinct characteristics and underlying mechanisms. By gaining insight into the different types of diabetes, you'll be better equipped to comprehend the nuances of your diagnosis.

Type 1 Diabetes: Unraveling the Immune System's Role

Type 1 diabetes is an autoimmune condition where the body's immune system mistakenly attacks and destroys the insulin-producing beta cells in the pancreas. This results in a severe insulin deficiency, requiring individuals to rely on insulin injections for life. Typically diagnosed in childhood or adolescence, type 1 diabetes accounts for approximately 5-10% of all diabetes cases.

Understanding the intricate dance between genetics and environmental triggers sheds light on why some individuals develop type 1 diabetes. Genetic predisposition plays a role, but environmental factors such as viral infections may trigger the autoimmune response leading to diabetes.

The management of type 1 diabetes involves a delicate balance of insulin administration, monitoring blood sugar levels, and adapting to lifestyle changes. The journey for individuals with type 1 diabetes is marked by resilience, as they navigate the complexities of insulin management while striving for a fulfilling life.

Type 2 Diabetes: Lifestyle Factors and Insulin Resistance

Type 2 diabetes, on the other hand, is characterized by insulin resistance and relative insulin deficiency. It is the most common form of diabetes, representing around 90-95% of all cases. Unlike type 1, type 2 diabetes is often associated with lifestyle factors such as poor diet, sedentary behavior, and obesity. Genetic factors also play a role, in influencing an individual's susceptibility to insulin resistance.

Insulin resistance occurs when cells in the body no longer respond effectively to insulin, leading to elevated blood sugar levels. Over time, the pancreas may struggle to produce enough insulin to overcome this resistance, resulting in type 2 diabetes.

Managing type 2 diabetes involves lifestyle modifications, including dietary changes, increased physical activity, and, in some cases, oral medications or insulin therapy. Empowering individuals with the knowledge and tools to make healthier choices is a central aspect of type 2 diabetes management.

Gestational Diabetes: Navigating Pregnancy-Related Challenges

Gestational diabetes is a unique type that occurs during pregnancy. While temporary, it requires careful management to protect the health of both the mother and the developing baby. Hormonal changes during pregnancy can lead to insulin resistance, and in some cases, the pancreas may struggle to produce enough insulin.

Managing gestational diabetes involves close monitoring of blood sugar levels, dietary adjustments, and, in some cases, insulin therapy. While gestational diabetes typically resolves after childbirth, it raises the risk of developing type 2 diabetes later in life for both the mother and the child.

LADA and Other Forms: Exploring Variations

Beyond the more commonly known types, there are variations such as Latent Autoimmune Diabetes in Adults (LADA) and other rare forms of diabetes. LADA shares similarities with both type 1 and type 2 diabetes, often appearing in adulthood with a gradual onset of autoimmune destruction of beta cells.

Exploring these variations contributes to a deeper understanding of the heterogeneity within the diabetes spectrum. Recognizing the distinctions allows for tailored approaches to management, acknowledging that each individual's journey with diabetes is unique.

Understanding the different types of diabetes involves unraveling the intricate interplay of genetics, immune responses, and lifestyle factors. By appreciating the distinctions between type 1, type 2, gestational diabetes, and other variations, you pave the way for informed decision-making and proactive management of your diabetes journey.

The Underlying Causes of Diabetes

To comprehend diabetes fully, it is essential to delve into the underlying causes that set the stage for this complex condition. Diabetes is not a singular entity with a single cause; rather, it emerges from a convergence of genetic, environmental, and lifestyle factors. Exploring these contributing factors will provide you with a more holistic perspective on the roots of diabetes.

Genetic Predisposition: The Role of Inherited Traits

Genetics plays a significant role in diabetes susceptibility. Individuals with a family history of diabetes are at a higher risk, indicating a hereditary component. While not everyone with a family history will develop diabetes, genetic predisposition can influence the likelihood of its occurrence.

Numerous genes associated with diabetes risk have been identified, affecting various aspects of insulin production, insulin action, and glucose metabolism. Understanding your genetic predisposition can offer valuable insights into your risk profile and guide proactive measures to mitigate potential risks.

Environmental Triggers: Unraveling External Influences

While genetics sets the stage, environmental factors often act as triggers that initiate the onset of diabetes, particularly in genetically predisposed individuals. Viral infections, for example, have been implicated in triggering the autoimmune response leading to type 1 diabetes.

Moreover, lifestyle factors such as diet, physical activity, and exposure to stress contribute significantly to the development of type 2 diabetes. Diets high in refined sugars and saturated fats, combined with sedentary lifestyles, can contribute to obesity and insulin resistance, key factors in the development of type 2 diabetes.

Autoimmune Responses: When the Body Turns Against Itself

In type 1 diabetes, the immune system plays a central role. It mistakenly identifies the insulin-producing beta cells in the pancreas as foreign invaders and launches an autoimmune attack, leading to the destruction of these crucial cells.

Understanding the intricacies of autoimmune responses in diabetes is a dynamic area of research. Unraveling the specific triggers that initiate the autoimmune cascade holds promise for future therapeutic interventions aimed at halting or preventing the progression of type 1 diabetes.

Insulin Resistance: The Core Mechanism of Type 2 Diabetes

Type 2 diabetes revolves around the concept of insulin resistance, where the body's cells become less responsive to the effects of insulin. Initially, the pancreas compensates by producing more insulin, but over time, this compensatory mechanism falters, leading to elevated blood sugar levels.

The factors contributing to insulin resistance are multifaceted and include genetics, obesity, sedentary behavior, and certain medical conditions. By addressing these factors, individuals with type 2 diabetes can improve insulin sensitivity and better manage their condition.

Lifestyle Factors: The Intersection of Choices and Health

Perhaps one of the most impactful determinants of diabetes is lifestyle. The choices we make regarding our diet, physical activity, and stress management directly influence our risk of developing diabetes. A diet rich in whole foods, regular physical activity, and effective stress management can significantly reduce the risk of type 2 diabetes.

Educating individuals about the profound impact of lifestyle choices empowers them to take control of their health. Small, sustainable changes in daily habits can yield substantial benefits, not only in diabetes prevention but also in the management of the condition for those already diagnosed.

In essence, the underlying causes of diabetes are a dynamic interplay of genetic predisposition, environmental triggers, autoimmune responses, insulin resistance, and lifestyle factors. By comprehensively understanding these factors, you gain valuable insights into the complexities of diabetes and pave the way for proactive and informed management.

Recognizing the Common Symptoms of Diabetes

Recognizing the symptoms of diabetes is the first step toward early detection and effective management. While the specific symptoms may vary among different types of diabetes, there are common signs that serve as red flags, prompting further investigation and evaluation. By familiarizing yourself with these symptoms, you become an active participant in your health, enabling timely intervention and improved outcomes.

Frequent Urination and Excessive Thirst: The Telltale Signs of High Blood Sugar

One of the hallmark symptoms of diabetes is polyuria or frequent urination. When blood sugar levels are elevated, the kidneys work overtime to filter and excrete the excess glucose, leading to increased urine production. This, in turn, triggers excessive thirst as the body attempts to compensate for fluid loss.

Recognizing changes in your urinary habits, such as needing to urinate more frequently, and experiencing unquenchable thirst, should prompt further investigation, especially if these symptoms are persistent.

Unexplained Weight Loss: A Warning Sign for Diabetes

Unexplained weight loss can be an early indicator of diabetes, particularly in cases of type 1 diabetes. When the body cannot effectively use glucose for energy due to insulin deficiency, it begins to break down muscle and fat for fuel. This metabolic shift can result in noticeable and unintentional weight loss.

If you find yourself losing weight without making intentional changes to your diet or activity level, it's essential to consider the possibility of diabetes and seek medical evaluation.

Increased Hunger: The Paradox of Insufficient Fuel

While unexplained weight loss is a common symptom, increased hunger can paradoxically accompany diabetes. When cells are unable to utilize glucose effectively, the body perceives a shortage of energy, leading to heightened feelings of hunger.

Experiencing persistent and unexplained hunger, especially in conjunction with other symptoms, warrants attention and further investigation to rule out or confirm diabetes.

Fatigue and Weakness: The Impact of Unregulated Blood Sugar

The fluctuations in blood sugar levels characteristic of diabetes can contribute to feelings of fatigue and weakness. When cells lack sufficient glucose for energy due to insulin-related issues, the body's overall energy levels can plummet, leading to persistent tiredness.

If you find yourself constantly fatigued, despite getting adequate rest, it's crucial to explore potential underlying causes, with diabetes being one of them.

Blurred Vision: Unmasking the Impact on Eye Health

Vision changes, particularly blurred vision, can be associated with diabetes. High blood sugar levels can affect the fluid balance in the lenses of the eyes, leading to temporary changes in vision.

While blurred vision can have various causes, it is essential not to ignore this symptom, especially if it occurs alongside other diabetes-related signs.

Numbness or Tingling in Extremities: Unveiling Neuropathy

Diabetes can impact the nerves, leading to a condition known as neuropathy. Numbness or tingling sensations, particularly in the hands and feet, may indicate nerve damage associated with uncontrolled diabetes.

Recognizing and addressing neuropathic symptoms early is crucial to prevent further nerve damage and complications.

Slow-Healing Wounds and Frequent Infections: Indicators of Compromised Immunity

Diabetes can compromise the immune system, making individuals more susceptible to infections. Slow-healing wounds and frequent infections, particularly in the skin and urinary tract, can be indicative of underlying diabetes.

Monitoring the healing process of wounds and addressing recurrent infections promptly is essential for overall health management in individuals with diabetes.

Recognizing the common symptoms of diabetes involves paying attention to subtle changes in urinary habits, weight, hunger, energy levels, vision, and overall well-being. By being vigilant and proactive in seeking medical evaluation for persistent symptoms, you empower yourself to take control of your health and initiate timely interventions for effective diabetes management.

CHAPTER 2

Diagnosis and Initial Steps

Receiving a diabetes diagnosis marks the beginning of a transformative journey. In this chapter, we will delve into the diagnosis process, providing insights into what to expect, coping mechanisms for the initial shock, strategies for emotional well-being, and the importance of assembling a dedicated diabetes care team.

The Diagnosis Process: What to Expect

The journey from experiencing symptoms to receiving a diabetes diagnosis is a pivotal stage in your health narrative. Understanding the diagnosis process empowers you to navigate this phase with awareness and resilience.

Recognizing Symptoms: From Red Flags to Seeking Answers

The first step in the diagnosis process often begins with recognizing symptoms that may indicate diabetes. As discussed in the previous chapter, symptoms such as frequent urination, excessive thirst, unexplained weight loss, and fatigue can serve as red flags.

When these symptoms become noticeable and persistent, it's crucial to seek medical attention promptly. Your primary care physician will likely conduct initial screenings, including blood tests, to assess your blood sugar levels and determine if further evaluation for diabetes is necessary.

Diagnostic Blood Tests: Unraveling the Numbers

Blood tests are fundamental to the diagnosis of diabetes. The most common diagnostic tests include fasting blood sugar tests, oral glucose tolerance tests, and HbA1c tests. Each test provides different insights into your blood sugar levels, helping healthcare professionals make an accurate diagnosis.

The fasting blood sugar test measures your blood sugar level after an overnight fast. Elevated fasting blood sugar levels may indicate diabetes. The oral glucose tolerance test involves fasting overnight and then consuming a sugary solution. Blood sugar levels are tested at intervals to assess how your body processes glucose. An HbA1c test provides a snapshot of your average blood sugar levels over the past two to three months.

Understanding the results of these tests is a crucial aspect of the diagnosis process. Elevated blood sugar levels may prompt further evaluation, including additional tests and discussions about your medical history and lifestyle factors.

Confirmatory Tests and Further Evaluation

In some cases, additional tests may be necessary to confirm a diabetes diagnosis and determine the specific type. These tests may include antibody tests to check for autoimmune activity in the case of type 1 diabetes or C-peptide tests to assess insulin production.

Further evaluation involves discussions with your healthcare provider about your symptoms, medical history, and lifestyle factors. This holistic approach ensures a comprehensive understanding of your health and facilitates tailored recommendations for management.

Receiving a diabetes diagnosis is a pivotal moment, and the information gathered during the diagnosis process lays the foundation for informed decision-making and proactive management of your health.

Coping with the Initial Shock

The moment you receive a diabetes diagnosis can be an emotional whirlwind. Coping with the initial shock requires a combination of self-awareness, support from loved ones, and a proactive mindset. Let's explore strategies to navigate this phase with resilience and empowerment.

Acknowledging Your Emotions: It's Okay to Feel

Upon receiving a diabetes diagnosis, it's natural to experience a range of emotions. Shock, disbelief, fear, and even grief for the perceived loss of normalcy are all valid responses. It's essential to acknowledge and validate these emotions without judgment.

Allow yourself the space to feel and process your emotions. This is not a sign of weakness but a crucial step in adapting to the new reality. Reach out to supportive friends or family members who can lend a listening ear and provide comfort during this initial phase.

Education as Empowerment: Understanding Your Condition

Knowledge is a powerful tool for coping with the shock of a diabetes diagnosis. Take the time to educate yourself about diabetes—its types, causes, and management strategies. Understanding the condition empowers you to actively participate in your own health and treatment decisions.

Your healthcare provider is a valuable resource for information. Ask questions, seek clarification, and express any concerns you may have. The more informed you are about diabetes, the better equipped you'll be to navigate the challenges and make decisions aligned with your health goals.

Building a Support System: You Are Not Alone

Coping with the shock of a diabetes diagnosis is not a solitary journey. Building a strong support system is essential for emotional well-being. Share your diagnosis with trusted friends, family members, or support groups who can offer encouragement, understanding, and practical assistance.

Having a support system provides a network of individuals who can accompany you on this journey, offering emotional support during challenging times and celebrating your successes. Joining diabetes support groups, either in person or online, can connect you with others who share similar experiences and insights.

Shifting Perspectives: From Challenge to Opportunity

While the initial shock of a diabetes diagnosis may feel overwhelming, it's essential to shift perspectives and view this as an opportunity for positive change. Embrace the opportunity to adopt a healthier lifestyle, make informed choices about your diet and physical activity, and prioritize self-care.

Focus on the aspects of your life that you can control. Small, incremental changes can lead to significant improvements in your overall well-being. By reframing the diagnosis as a catalyst for positive transformation, you take an active role in shaping your health journey.

In essence, coping with the initial shock of a diabetes diagnosis involves acknowledging your emotions, educating yourself about the condition, building a strong support system, and shifting your perspective towards empowerment and positive change.

Emotional well-being is an integral aspect of living well with diabetes. Developing effective coping strategies is essential for navigating the emotional challenges that may arise after receiving a diabetes diagnosis. Let's explore practical and empowering strategies for emotional coping.

Mindfulness and Stress Reduction: Nurturing Inner Calm

Mindfulness practices, such as meditation and deep breathing exercises, can be powerful tools for managing stress and promoting emotional well-being. These practices encourage you to stay present in the moment, fostering a sense of calm and centeredness.

Incorporate mindfulness into your daily routine, even if only for a few minutes. Whether through guided meditation apps, deep-breathing exercises, or moments of quiet reflection, mindfulness can help alleviate stress and enhance your overall emotional resilience.

Journaling: Processing Thoughts and Emotions

Keeping a journal provides a safe space to express your thoughts and emotions. Documenting your journey with diabetes, including your challenges, triumphs, and reflections, can be therapeutic. Journaling allows you to process complex emotions, gain insights into patterns of behavior, and track your progress over time.

Consider starting a diabetes journal where you record your daily experiences, emotions, and any notable events related to your health. Reflecting on your entries can offer a deeper understanding of your emotional landscape and provide a tool for self-discovery.

Seeking Professional Support: Therapy and Counseling

The emotional impact of a diabetes diagnosis may benefit from professional support. Therapists, counselors, or psychologists with experience in chronic conditions can offer valuable insights and coping strategies tailored to your individual needs.

Professional support provides a confidential space to explore the emotional aspects of living with diabetes. It can help you develop resilience, coping mechanisms, and a positive mindset as you navigate the challenges and adjustments associated with the condition.

Connecting with Others: Shared Experiences and Understanding

Engaging with others who share similar experiences can foster a sense of connection and understanding. Diabetes support groups, whether in-person or online, provide a platform to share insights, exchange coping strategies, and receive encouragement from individuals who understand the unique challenges of living with diabetes.

Sharing your own experiences can be empowering not only for you but also for others facing similar journeys. Establishing connections with individuals who have walked a similar path reinforces the notion that you are not alone and that there is a supportive community ready to share insights and offer encouragement.

Setting Realistic Goals: Celebrating Progress

Emotional well-being is closely tied to a sense of accomplishment and progress. Setting realistic goals, both short-term and long-term, provides a roadmap for your diabetes management journey. Celebrate even the smallest achievements, as each step forward contributes to your overall well-being.

Consider creating a list of achievable goals related to your health, lifestyle, or emotional resilience. Regularly reassess and adjust these goals based on your evolving needs and experiences. By acknowledging and celebrating your progress, you reinforce a positive and proactive mindset.

Emotional coping strategies for the newly diagnosed involve mindfulness practices, journaling, seeking professional support, connecting with others, and setting realistic goals. Integrating these strategies into your daily life fosters emotional resilience and empowers you to navigate the emotional complexities of living with diabetes.

Assembling Your Diabetes Care Team

Managing diabetes is not a solo endeavor; it requires a collaborative approach involving a dedicated diabetes care team. Assembling a team of healthcare professionals ensures comprehensive and personalized care, addressing both the medical and emotional aspects of living with diabetes.

Primary Care Physician: Your Central Point of Contact

Your primary care physician plays a central role in your diabetes care team. They are often the first point of contact during the diagnosis process and remain a key collaborator in managing your overall health. Regular check-ups with your primary care physician involve monitoring blood sugar levels, assessing overall health, and addressing any emerging concerns.

Developing a strong and open relationship with your primary care physician fosters effective communication and ensures that your diabetes management aligns with your broader healthcare needs.

Endocrinologist: Specialized Diabetes Care

An endocrinologist, a healthcare professional specializing in hormonal disorders, is a crucial member of your diabetes care team. Endocrinologists have specific expertise in diabetes management and can provide in-depth insights into insulin therapy, medication adjustments, and long-term strategies for diabetes control.

Consulting with an endocrinologist ensures that your diabetes management plan is tailored to your individual needs. They may also collaborate with other specialists as needed, creating a comprehensive and integrated approach to your care.

Diabetes Educator: Empowering Your Knowledge

A diabetes educator plays a vital role in empowering you with the knowledge and skills needed to manage your diabetes effectively. These healthcare professionals provide education on topics such as blood sugar monitoring, medication management, and lifestyle modifications.

Engaging with a diabetes educator enhances your understanding of the practical aspects of diabetes management. They can guide you in making informed decisions and navigating the day-to-day challenges associated with living with diabetes.

Registered Dietitian: Tailoring Nutritional Guidance

Nutrition is a cornerstone of diabetes management, and a registered dietitian is an essential member of your care team. These professionals specialize in providing personalized nutritional guidance based on your unique health needs and goals.

Working with a registered dietitian involves developing a balanced meal plan, understanding carbohydrate counting, and making informed food choices that align with your diabetes management plan. Their expertise contributes to overall health and well-being.

Pharmacist: Medication Management Expertise

A pharmacist is a valuable resource for understanding and managing your diabetes medications. They can provide insights into proper medication administration, potential side effects, and interactions with other medications. Regular communication with your pharmacist ensures that you are well informed about your medications and can address any concerns or questions that may arise.

Podiatrist: Foot Health and Diabetes

Foot care is a crucial aspect of diabetes management, and a podiatrist specializes in the health of your feet. Diabetes can impact circulation and nerve function in the feet, increasing the risk of complications. Regular check-ups with a podiatrist help prevent and address any foot-related issues, reducing the risk of more serious complications.

Psychologist or Counselor: Emotional Well-Being Support

The emotional impact of living with diabetes necessitates the inclusion of a psychologist or counselor in your care team. These professionals specialize in providing emotional support, coping strategies, and mental health guidance. Managing the emotional aspects of diabetes is integral to overall well-being, and a psychologist or counselor can offer valuable insights and coping tools.

Assembling your diabetes care team involves collaborating with healthcare professionals who specialize in different aspects of diabetes management. From your primary care physician and endocrinologist to diabetes educators, dietitians, pharmacists, podiatrists, and mental health professionals, each member plays a unique role in ensuring comprehensive and personalized care. Establishing a strong and collaborative relationship with your care team is foundational to successfully managing your diabetes and living a healthy, fulfilling life.

CHAPTER 3

Blood Sugar Monitoring and Management

Living well with diabetes requires active and informed management of blood sugar levels. In this chapter, we will delve into the significance of regular blood sugar monitoring, explore the intricacies of glucose levels and target ranges, and guide you through the process of developing a personalized diabetes management plan.

The Importance of Regular Blood Sugar Monitoring

Regular blood sugar monitoring is a cornerstone of effective diabetes management. It provides essential insights into how your body processes glucose, allowing you to make informed decisions about your lifestyle, medication, and overall well-being.

Understanding Blood Sugar Dynamics: The Role of Glucose in the Body

To appreciate the importance of blood sugar monitoring, it's essential to understand the role of glucose in the body. Glucose is a primary source of energy for cells, and its levels are tightly regulated to ensure optimal bodily functions.

When you eat, the carbohydrates in food are broken down into glucose, which enters the bloodstream. In response, the pancreas releases insulin, a hormone that facilitates the uptake of glucose by cells for energy. In individuals with diabetes, this intricate balance is disrupted, leading to elevated blood sugar levels.

The Impact of Uncontrolled Blood Sugar: Short-Term and Long-Term Consequences

Uncontrolled blood sugar levels can have both immediate and long-term consequences. In the short term, high blood sugar can cause symptoms such as excessive thirst, frequent urination, fatigue, and blurred vision. If left untreated, it can progress to a serious condition known as diabetic ketoacidosis (DKA), which requires urgent medical attention.

Over the long term, uncontrolled diabetes can lead to a range of complications affecting the heart, kidneys, eyes, and nerves. These complications underscore the importance of proactive blood sugar monitoring to prevent and manage potential risks.

Empowering Self-Management: The Key to Successful Diabetes Care

Regular blood sugar monitoring empowers individuals with diabetes to take an active role in their self-management. It provides real-time feedback on the impact of dietary choices, physical activity, medication, and other factors on blood sugar levels.

By monitoring blood sugar levels regularly, you gain a deeper understanding of how your body responds to different inputs. This knowledge forms the basis for informed decision-making and allows you to make adjustments to your lifestyle and treatment plan as needed.

Individualized Insights: Recognizing Personal Patterns

Every person with diabetes is unique, and individual responses to various factors, such as meals, stress, and physical activity, can vary. Regular blood sugar monitoring helps you recognize personal patterns and trends, enabling you to tailor your diabetes management plan to your specific needs.

For example, you may notice that your blood sugar levels tend to spike after consuming certain foods. Armed with this knowledge, you can make informed choices about your diet, opting for alternatives that have a more favorable impact on your blood sugar levels.

In summary, the importance of regular blood sugar monitoring cannot be overstated. It empowers individuals with diabetes to actively manage their condition, prevent short-term complications, mitigate long-term risks, and gain personalized insights into their unique responses to various factors.

Understanding Glucose Levels and Target Ranges

Understanding glucose levels and target ranges is fundamental to effective diabetes management. This knowledge forms the basis for making informed decisions about medication, diet, and lifestyle. In this section, we will explore the dynamics of glucose levels, optimal target ranges, and the factors influencing these parameters.

Fasting Blood Sugar Levels: Establishing Baseline Measurements

Fasting blood sugar levels are typically measured in the morning before consuming food or drink. This measurement provides a baseline indication of how well your body maintains glucose levels during periods of fasting.

For individuals without diabetes, normal fasting blood sugar levels typically fall between 70 and 100 milligrams per deciliter (mg/dL). However, target ranges may vary based on individual health conditions, and it's essential to work with your healthcare provider to establish personalized targets.

Postprandial Blood Sugar Levels: Monitoring After Meals

Postprandial blood sugar levels refer to measurements taken after meals. These levels give insights into how effectively your body processes glucose from the food you've consumed. Postprandial targets may vary, but, in general, levels below 180 mg/dL two hours after meals are considered acceptable for many individuals with diabetes.

Monitoring postprandial blood sugar levels allows you to identify how different meals impact your glucose levels and make informed choices about portion sizes, meal composition, and timing.

HbA1c: A Measure of Long-Term Blood Sugar Control

HbA1c, or glycated hemoglobin, provides a snapshot of your average blood sugar levels over the past two to three months. This test is a valuable tool for assessing long-term blood sugar control and is often used to guide adjustments in diabetes management plans.

For individuals without diabetes, HbA1c levels typically fall below 5.7%. However, target ranges for individuals with diabetes may vary. Generally, an HbA1c level below 7% is considered acceptable, but individualized targets may be established based on factors such as age, overall health, and the presence of other medical conditions.

Continuous Glucose Monitoring (CGM): Real-Time Insights

Continuous Glucose Monitoring (CGM) systems provide real-time insights into blood sugar levels throughout the day and night. These devices use a tiny sensor inserted under the skin to measure glucose levels in the interstitial fluid.

CGM systems offer a more comprehensive view of blood sugar dynamics, allowing you to identify trends, patterns, and potential issues more effectively. They can be particularly beneficial for individuals who experience significant fluctuations in blood sugar levels.

Factors Influencing Glucose Levels: Beyond Food and Medication

While food and medication play central roles in influencing glucose levels, various other factors can impact blood sugar dynamics. Physical activity, stress, illness, and changes in routine can all influence how your body processes glucose.

Understanding how these factors affect your glucose levels enables you to make informed adjustments to your diabetes management plan. For example, if you know that stress tends to elevate your blood sugar levels, incorporating stress-reduction techniques into your routine becomes a proactive measure.

Setting Personalized Targets: Collaboration with Your Healthcare Team

Establishing personalized target ranges for blood sugar levels is a collaborative process involving you and your healthcare team. Your healthcare provider will consider factors such as your age, overall health, presence of other medical conditions, and individual preferences when setting targets.

Regular discussions with your healthcare provider allow you to review your blood sugar data, discuss any challenges or concerns, and make adjustments to your management plan as needed. This ongoing collaboration ensures that your targets align with your overall health goals and provide a realistic framework for successful diabetes management.

Understanding glucose levels and target ranges is integral to effective diabetes management. Fasting and postprandial measurements, HbA1c tests, continuous glucose monitoring, and awareness of influencing factors collectively contribute to a comprehensive understanding of blood sugar dynamics. By working closely with your healthcare team to set personalized targets, you empower yourself to make informed decisions that promote optimal blood sugar control and overall well-being.

Developing a Personalized Diabetes Management Plan

Developing a personalized diabetes management plan is a dynamic and collaborative process that involves various elements, from lifestyle adjustments to medication management. In this section, we will explore the key components of a personalized plan, emphasizing the importance of individualized approaches to diabetes care.

Holistic Assessment: Addressing Physical and Emotional Well-Being

A personalized diabetes management plan begins with a holistic assessment of your physical and emotional well-being. Your healthcare provider will consider factors such as your medical history, lifestyle, dietary habits, physical activity, stress levels, and emotional resilience.

This comprehensive assessment lays the foundation for tailoring your management plan to address your unique needs and goals. By considering both physical and emotional aspects, your healthcare team can create a plan that aligns with your overall well-being.

Diet and Nutrition: Crafting a Balanced Approach

Diet and nutrition play pivotal roles in diabetes management. A registered dietitian can work with you to create a balanced and personalized meal plan that aligns with your dietary preferences, cultural considerations, and health goals.

Emphasizing whole foods, managing portion sizes, and incorporating a variety of nutrient-dense foods contribute to stable blood sugar levels. Your dietitian will guide carbohydrate counting, food choices, and strategies for managing postprandial blood sugar levels effectively.

Physical Activity: Integrating Exercise Into Daily Life

Regular physical activity is a cornerstone of diabetes management, contributing to improved insulin sensitivity and overall health. Your healthcare team can help you develop an exercise plan tailored to your fitness level, preferences, and any existing health conditions.

Whether it's walking, cycling, swimming, or engaging in other forms of exercise, finding activities you enjoy enhances adherence to your plan. Establishing a routine that incorporates both aerobic and strength-training exercises contributes to optimal physical well-being.

Medication Management: Finding the Right Balance

For many individuals with diabetes, medication is a crucial component of their management plan. The type and dosage of medications prescribed will depend on the specific type of diabetes, individual health factors, and overall management goals.

Oral medications, insulin therapy, or a combination of both may be recommended. It's essential to work closely with your healthcare provider to understand the purpose of each medication, potential side effects, and strategies for proper administration.

Blood Sugar Monitoring: A Daily Practice

As discussed earlier, regular blood sugar monitoring is a fundamental aspect of diabetes management. Incorporating this practice into your daily routine provides insights into how your body responds to various factors, enabling you to make informed decisions about your lifestyle, diet, and medication.

Discuss with your healthcare provider the frequency and timing of blood sugar monitoring that best aligns with your individual needs. CGM systems or traditional fingerstick methods can be utilized, depending on your preferences and requirements.

Stress Management: Prioritizing Emotional Well-Being

The emotional aspects of living with diabetes should not be overlooked. Stress can impact blood sugar levels, and managing emotional well-being is integral to overall health. Integrating stress-reduction techniques, such as mindfulness, meditation, or counseling, into your routine contributes to a balanced and resilient mindset.

Regular check-ins with a psychologist or counselor provide a safe space to discuss emotional challenges, develop coping strategies, and address any concerns related to living with diabetes.

Regular Follow-Up: Adapting to Evolving Needs

A personalized diabetes management plan is not static; it evolves based on your changing needs, experiences, and health status. Regular follow-up appointments with your healthcare team provide opportunities to review your progress, discuss any challenges, and make adjustments to your plan as needed.

These follow-up sessions also allow you to stay informed about advancements in diabetes management, new technologies, and emerging treatment options. Staying actively engaged with your healthcare team ensures that your management plan remains aligned with your goals and the latest developments in diabetes care.

Collaboration with Your Diabetes Care Team: A Partnership for Success

The development and implementation of a personalized diabetes management plan are collaborative processes. Your active participation, open communication, and willingness to embrace lifestyle changes are essential elements of success.

Collaborate closely with your healthcare team, including your primary care physician, endocrinologist, diabetes educator, registered dietitian, and other specialists. Establishing a partnership based on trust, shared decision-making, and a mutual commitment to your well-being forms the foundation for effective diabetes management.

Developing a personalized diabetes management plan involves a holistic assessment of your physical and emotional well-being, addressing key components such as diet, physical activity, medication management, blood sugar monitoring, stress management, and regular follow-up. By actively collaborating with your healthcare team and embracing individualized approaches, you pave the way for successful diabetes management and a fulfilling, healthy life.

CHAPTER 4

Healthy Eating for Diabetes

Maintaining a well-balanced and nutritious diet is a cornerstone of effective diabetes management. In this chapter, we will explore the critical role of nutrition in managing diabetes, delve into the creation of a balanced meal plan, discuss the principles of carbohydrate counting and meal timing, and provide insights into making smart food choices that support overall health.

The Role of Nutrition in Diabetes Management

Understanding the role of nutrition is paramount for individuals living with diabetes. The food choices you make directly impact blood sugar levels, making nutrition a powerful tool for managing the condition. Let's explore the multifaceted role of nutrition in diabetes management.

Nutrition as a Cornerstone of Diabetes Management

Nutrition plays a central role in diabetes management, influencing blood sugar levels, insulin sensitivity, and overall well-being. The goal of a diabetes-friendly diet is to regulate blood sugar levels, maintain a healthy weight, and reduce the risk of complications associated with the condition.

Balanced nutrition provides the essential nutrients needed for optimal bodily functions, including carbohydrates, proteins, fats, vitamins, and minerals. Crafting a well-rounded diet involves making informed choices about the types and proportions of foods consumed.

Impact of Carbohydrates on Blood Sugar Levels

Carbohydrates have a direct and significant impact on blood sugar levels. When consumed, carbohydrates are broken down into glucose, leading to an increase in blood sugar. For individuals with diabetes, managing carbohydrate intake is a key aspect of controlling blood sugar levels.

Different carbohydrates have varying effects on blood sugar, with some causing rapid spikes and others leading to more gradual increases. Understanding the glycemic index (GI) of foods helps individuals make choices that minimize sudden surges in blood sugar.

Balancing Macronutrients: Carbohydrates, Proteins, and Fats

A well-balanced diet for diabetes management involves the thoughtful distribution of macronutrients—carbohydrates, proteins, and fats. Each macronutrient serves a unique purpose in supporting overall health, and finding the right balance is essential for optimal diabetes care.

- **Carbohydrates:** While controlling the quantity and quality of carbohydrates is crucial, they remain an essential energy source. Prioritizing complex carbohydrates, such as whole grains, legumes, and vegetables, over simple sugars helps regulate blood sugar levels more effectively.

- **Proteins:** Protein is vital for maintaining muscle mass, supporting immune function, and promoting overall satiety. Sources of lean protein, such as poultry, fish, tofu, and legumes, can be incorporated into meals to enhance nutritional balance.

- **Fats:** Including healthy fats in the diet is essential for heart health and overall well-being. Opt for unsaturated fats found in sources like avocados, nuts, seeds, and olive oil while moderating saturated and trans fats to promote cardiovascular health.

Caloric Intake and Weight Management

Maintaining a healthy weight is a key component of diabetes management. Caloric intake should be aligned with individual energy needs to prevent weight gain or loss. For those aiming to lose weight, a gradual and sustainable approach is recommended, emphasizing a balanced diet and regular physical activity.

A registered dietitian can assist in determining appropriate caloric intake based on factors such as age, gender, activity level, and overall health. Tailoring caloric goals to individual needs ensures that nutritional requirements are met while supporting weight management goals.

The role of nutrition in diabetes management extends beyond controlling blood sugar levels. A well-balanced diet supports overall health, helps manage weight, and provides essential nutrients for optimal bodily functions. Understanding the impact of carbohydrates, balancing macronutrients, and managing caloric intake are fundamental principles that guide effective nutrition for individuals with diabetes.

Creating a Balanced Meal Plan

Crafting a balanced meal plan is a practical and effective approach to managing diabetes. A well-designed meal plan considers nutritional needs, portion control, and the distribution of macronutrients throughout the day. Let's explore the key elements of creating a balanced meal plan for diabetes management.

Meal Planning Basics: Building a Foundation for Success

Effective meal planning involves thoughtful consideration of portion sizes, food choices, and the timing of meals. Creating a foundation for success begins with a few fundamental principles:

- **Consistent Meal Timing:** Establishing regular meal times helps regulate blood sugar levels and supports the effectiveness of medication or insulin. Aim for three main meals per day with well-timed snacks if needed.

- **Balanced Plate Method:** The plate method is a visual guide for creating balanced meals. Fill half of your plate with non-starchy vegetables, one quarter with lean protein, and one-quarter with whole grains or starchy vegetables. Adding a serving of fruit and a source of healthy fat completes the balanced plate.

- **Portion Control:** Monitoring portion sizes is essential for managing caloric intake and blood sugar levels. Measuring food portions, using smaller plates, and being mindful of serving sizes contribute to effective portion control.

Carbohydrate Counting: Precision in Blood Sugar Management

Carbohydrate counting is a valuable tool for individuals with diabetes, allowing for precise management of blood sugar levels. By tracking the number of carbohydrates consumed, individuals can make informed decisions about insulin dosages, medication, and meal composition.

- **Understanding Carbohydrate Sources:** Different foods contribute varying amounts of carbohydrates. It's essential to recognize carbohydrate sources, including grains, fruits, dairy products, and legumes, and be mindful of their impact on blood sugar levels.

- **Carbohydrate Counting Techniques:** Carbohydrate counting can be approached in various ways, including counting grams of carbohydrates, using food exchange lists, or utilizing smartphone apps that assist in tracking nutritional content. The chosen method should align with individual preferences and lifestyle.

- **Adjusting Insulin or Medication:** For individuals using insulin or certain medications, carbohydrate counting facilitates precise adjustments. Understanding the carbohydrate content of meals allows for more accurate dosing, promoting optimal blood sugar control.

Incorporating Nutrient-Dense Foods: A Focus on Whole Foods

A balanced meal plan emphasizes nutrient-dense foods that provide essential vitamins, minerals, and fiber. Choosing whole foods over processed options supports overall health and aids in blood sugar management.

- **Fruits and Vegetables:** Incorporate a variety of colorful fruits and vegetables into meals. These foods are rich in fiber, antioxidants, and essential nutrients. Aim to fill half of your plate with non-starchy vegetables to promote satiety and nutritional balance.

- **Whole Grains:** Opt for whole grains such as brown rice, quinoa, oats, and whole wheat bread instead of refined grains. Whole grains contain fiber, which helps regulate blood sugar levels and promotes digestive health.

- **Lean Proteins:** Include lean protein sources in your meals to support muscle health and enhance satiety.

Options such as poultry, fish, tofu, legumes, and low-fat dairy products contribute to a well-rounded and satisfying diet.

- **Healthy Fats:** Incorporate sources of healthy fats, such as avocados, nuts, seeds, and olive oil, into your meals. These fats contribute to heart health and add flavor and texture to dishes.

Hydration: The Overlooked Component of Nutrition

Proper hydration is often overlooked but is a crucial component of overall nutrition and diabetes management. Water supports various bodily functions, helps control appetite, and aids in digestion.

- **Water Intake Guidelines:** The general recommendation for daily water intake is around 8 cups (64 ounces) for most adults. However, individual needs may vary based on factors such as age, activity level, and climate.

- **Balancing Beverages:** Be mindful of beverage choices, as some may contain added sugars or contribute to excessive calorie intake. Water, herbal teas, and other low-calorie options are preferable choices for hydration.

Carbohydrate Counting and Meal Timing

Precision in carbohydrate counting and meal timing is essential for effective blood sugar management in diabetes. Understanding the impact of carbohydrates, planning meals with balanced macronutrients, and considering the timing of meals contribute to optimal glucose control.

The Significance of Carbohydrate Counting

Carbohydrate counting is a valuable strategy for individuals with diabetes to manage blood sugar levels effectively. By quantifying the amount of carbohydrates in meals, individuals can make informed decisions about insulin doses, medication, and overall dietary choices.

- **Carbohydrate Impact on Blood Sugar:** Carbohydrates have a direct impact on blood sugar levels, making them a crucial focus for individuals with diabetes. Different types of carbohydrates, such as simple sugars and complex carbohydrates, can have varying effects on blood sugar.

- **Tools for Carbohydrate Counting:** Various tools can assist in carbohydrate counting, including food labels, nutritional apps, and food scales. Familiarity with common serving sizes and portion control is essential for accurate carbohydrate counting.

- **Precision in Insulin Dosing:** For individuals using insulin, precise carbohydrate counting enables accurate insulin dosing. Understanding the carbohydrate content of meals allows for adjustments that align with individual insulin-to-carbohydrate ratios.

Balancing Macronutrients for Optimal Meal Planning

In addition to carbohydrate counting, balancing macronutrients—carbohydrates, proteins, and fats—contributes to well-rounded and satisfying meals. Each macronutrient plays a unique role in supporting overall health and blood sugar management.

- **Proteins for Satiety:** Including lean protein sources in meals promotes satiety and helps control appetite. Protein-rich foods, such as poultry, fish, tofu, and legumes, contribute to a balanced diet.

- **Healthy Fats for Flavor and Texture:** Incorporating healthy fats, such as avocados, nuts, seeds, and olive oil, adds flavor and texture to meals. Fats contribute to satiety and can help stabilize blood sugar levels when consumed in moderation.

- **Fiber for Digestive Health:** Foods rich in fiber, such as fruits, vegetables, and whole grains, contribute to digestive health and help regulate blood sugar levels. Including fiber in meals supports overall well-being.

Meal Timing and Blood Sugar Control

The timing of meals plays a significant role in blood sugar control. Establishing a regular meal schedule, spacing meals throughout the day, and considering the timing of snacks contribute to stable blood sugar levels.

- **Regular Meal Times:** Consistent meal times help regulate blood sugar levels by aligning with the body's natural rhythm. Aim for three main meals per day with well-timed snacks if needed.

- **Avoiding Prolonged Periods of Fasting:** Prolonged periods between meals can lead to fluctuations in blood sugar levels. Incorporating healthy snacks between meals helps maintain stable glucose levels and prevents overeating at subsequent meals.

- **Considering Physical Activity:** Meal timing can be coordinated with physical activity to optimize blood sugar management. Consuming a balanced meal or snack before exercise provides energy, while post-exercise nutrition aids in recovery.

The Role of Glycemic Index (GI) in Meal Planning

The glycemic index (GI) measures how quickly carbohydrates in foods raise blood sugar levels. While not the sole determinant of a food's healthfulness, understanding the GI can guide food choices for individuals with diabetes.

- **Low-GI Foods for Gradual Impact:** Low-GI foods, such as whole grains, legumes, and non-starchy vegetables, have a more gradual impact on blood sugar levels. Including these foods in meals supports stable glucose control.

- **Moderation of High-GI Foods:** High-GI foods, such as sugary snacks and refined grains, can cause rapid spikes in blood sugar. Consuming these foods in moderation and pairing them with sources of fiber and protein helps mitigate their impact.

- **Combining Foods for Balanced Effects:** Combining foods with varying GI values in a single meal can create a balanced overall impact on blood sugar levels. Pairing carbohydrates with proteins and fats can help slow the absorption of glucose.

Carbohydrate counting, balancing macronutrients, considering meal timing, and understanding the glycemic index are integral components of effective diabetes management. These strategies empower individuals to make informed decisions about their diet, optimize blood sugar control, and support overall well-being.

Making smart food choices is a key aspect of maintaining a healthy diet for individuals with diabetes. By prioritizing nutrient-dense foods, considering portion sizes, and being mindful of the impact of different food choices on blood sugar levels, individuals can optimize their nutrition for diabetes management.

Prioritizing Nutrient-Dense Foods

Nutrient-dense foods provide essential vitamins, minerals, and fiber without excess calories. Prioritizing these foods supports overall health, helps manage weight, and contributes to optimal blood sugar control.

- **Colorful Fruits and Vegetables:** Incorporate a variety of colorful fruits and vegetables into your diet. These foods are rich in antioxidants, vitamins, and fiber. Aim to fill half of your plate with non-starchy vegetables for a nutrient boost.

- **Lean Proteins:** Choose lean protein sources, such as poultry, fish, tofu, legumes, and low-fat dairy products. Protein is essential for muscle health, satiety, and overall well-being.

- **Whole Grains:** Opt for whole grains, such as brown rice, quinoa, oats, and whole wheat bread. Whole grains provide fiber, which supports digestive health and helps regulate blood sugar levels.

- **Healthy Fats:** Include sources of healthy fats, such as avocados, nuts, seeds, and olive oil, in your diet. These fats contribute to heart health and add flavor and texture to meals.

- **Dairy or Dairy Alternatives:** Choose low-fat or fat-free dairy products or dairy alternatives. These foods provide essential nutrients such as calcium and vitamin D without excessive saturated fat.

Considering Portion Sizes and Moderation

Portion control is crucial for managing caloric intake and blood sugar levels. Being mindful of portion sizes and practicing moderation allows individuals with diabetes to enjoy a variety of foods without compromising their health.

- **Use of Smaller Plates:** Using smaller plates can help control portion sizes and prevent overeating. The visual cues of a full plate contribute to a satisfying meal experience.

- **Listening to Hunger and Fullness Cues:** Pay attention to hunger and fullness cues to avoid overeating. Eating slowly, savoring each bite, and stopping when satisfied contribute to mindful eating.

- **Snacking with Purpose:** If snacking is part of your routine, choose nutrient-dense snacks and be mindful of portion sizes. Healthy snacks can contribute to overall nutrition and help manage blood sugar levels between meals.

- **Limiting Highly Processed Foods:** Highly processed foods often contain added sugars, unhealthy fats, and excessive calories. Limiting the intake of these foods supports overall health and diabetes management.

Understanding the Impact of Food Choices on Blood Sugar

Different foods have varying effects on blood sugar levels. Understanding the impact of food choices allows individuals with diabetes to make informed decisions about their diet and optimize blood sugar control.

- **Monitoring Carbohydrate Intake:** Carbohydrates have the most direct impact on blood sugar levels. Monitoring carbohydrate intake, especially from sources with a high glycemic index, helps regulate blood sugar.

- **Balancing Carbohydrates with Proteins and Fats:** Pairing carbohydrates with sources of protein and healthy fats can slow the absorption of glucose and reduce the overall impact on blood sugar levels.

- **Testing Blood Sugar Responses:** Individuals with diabetes can monitor their blood sugar responses to different foods. Keeping a food diary and noting blood sugar levels can provide valuable insights into the effects of specific foods on individual physiology.

- **Individualized Responses to Foods:** Each person may have unique responses to different foods. Factors such as genetics, metabolism, and overall health influence how the body processes and reacts to various nutrients.

Making Informed Choices in Various Settings

Making smart food choices extends beyond home-cooked meals to various settings, including restaurants, social gatherings, and travel. By planning, being aware of menu options, and making mindful choices, individuals with diabetes can navigate different environments successfully.

- **Restaurant Dining:** When dining out, consider reviewing the menu in advance, choosing grilled or baked options, and being mindful of portion sizes. Asking for sauces and dressings on the side allows for better control of added sugars and fats.

- **Social Gatherings:** Social events often involve a variety of food choices. Planning ahead, eating a balanced snack before the event, and being selective about food choices can help manage blood sugar levels during gatherings.

- **Traveling:** Traveling may present challenges in accessing familiar foods and maintaining regular meal times. Planning for snacks, staying hydrated, and having a supply of diabetes-friendly foods can help individuals manage their nutrition while on the go.

Seeking Guidance from Healthcare Professionals

Individuals with diabetes can benefit from seeking guidance from healthcare professionals, including registered dietitians and diabetes educators. These professionals can provide personalized advice, support dietary choices, and help individuals navigate the complexities of nutrition for diabetes management.

- **Registered Dietitian Support:** A registered dietitian specializing in diabetes care can offer tailored meal plans, carbohydrate counting guidance, and ongoing support. Working collaboratively with a dietitian ensures that nutrition plans align with individual health goals.

- **Diabetes Educator Insights:** Diabetes educators provide education on various aspects of diabetes management, including nutrition. They can offer practical tips, answer questions, and empower individuals to make informed choices about their diet.

Making smart food choices is a fundamental aspect of maintaining a healthy and balanced diet for individuals with diabetes. Prioritizing nutrient-dense foods, considering portion sizes, understanding the impact of food choices on blood sugar, and seeking guidance from healthcare professionals collectively contribute to effective nutrition management for individuals living with diabetes.

CHAPTER 5

Physical Activity and Exercise

Physical activity and exercise are integral components of a healthy lifestyle for individuals with diabetes. In this chapter, we will explore the numerous benefits of exercise for diabetes control, guide you in designing a personalized exercise routine that suits your needs, and provide insights into managing blood sugar effectively during physical activity.

Benefits of Exercise for Diabetes Control

Engaging in regular physical activity offers a multitude of benefits for individuals with diabetes. From improved blood sugar control to enhanced overall well-being, the positive impact of exercise is profound. Let's delve into the specific advantages that exercise brings to diabetes management.

Blood Sugar Regulation: Enhancing Insulin Sensitivity

One of the primary benefits of regular exercise is its positive effect on insulin sensitivity. Insulin is a hormone that facilitates the uptake of glucose by cells, and individuals with diabetes often experience reduced sensitivity to insulin. By engaging in physical activity, your body becomes more efficient at using insulin, leading to better blood sugar regulation.

- **Improved Glucose Uptake:** Exercise stimulates muscle cells to take up glucose from the bloodstream, reducing elevated blood sugar levels. This enhanced glucose uptake is particularly beneficial for individuals with insulin resistance.

- **Reduced Insulin Resistance:** Regular physical activity has been shown to reduce insulin resistance, a key factor in the development and progression of type 2 diabetes. Increased insulin sensitivity improves the body's ability to utilize glucose effectively.

Weight Management: Supporting Healthy Body Weight

Maintaining a healthy body weight is crucial for diabetes management, and exercise plays a pivotal role in achieving and sustaining weight goals. Physical activity contributes to calorie expenditure, promoting weight loss or weight maintenance, depending on individual needs.

- **Caloric Expenditure:** Exercise helps burn calories, supporting weight loss when combined with a balanced diet. For those at a healthy weight, regular physical activity aids in weight maintenance, preventing fluctuations that may impact blood sugar levels.

- **Muscle Mass Preservation:** Resistance training and weight-bearing exercises contribute to the preservation of muscle mass. As muscle tissue burns more calories than fat tissue, maintaining or increasing muscle mass supports a healthy metabolism.

Cardiovascular Health: Reducing Risk Factors

Individuals with diabetes are at an increased risk of cardiovascular complications. Exercise is a powerful ally in promoting heart health, and reducing risk factors such as high blood pressure and cholesterol levels.

- **Lowering Blood Pressure:** Regular physical activity has been shown to lower blood pressure, a critical factor in reducing the risk of heart disease and stroke. The cardiovascular benefits of exercise extend beyond blood sugar control.

- **Improving Lipid Profiles:** Exercise helps raise levels of high-density lipoprotein (HDL) cholesterol, often referred to as "good" cholesterol. Additionally, it can lower levels of low-density lipoprotein (LDL) cholesterol and triglycerides, further supporting cardiovascular health.

Enhanced Mood and Mental Well-Being

The positive impact of exercise extends beyond physical health to mental well-being. Engaging in regular physical activity has been linked to improved mood, reduced stress levels, and enhanced cognitive function.

- **Release of Endorphins:** Exercise triggers the release of endorphins, often referred to as "feel-good" hormones. These neurotransmitters contribute to a sense of well-being and can act as natural mood elevators.

- **Stress Reduction:** Physical activity is a known stress reliever, helping to reduce the physiological and psychological effects of stress. Managing stress is particularly important for individuals with diabetes, as stress can impact blood sugar levels.

- **Cognitive Benefits:** Exercise has been associated with improved cognitive function and a reduced risk of cognitive decline. Maintaining mental sharpness is essential for overall health and quality of life.

Enhanced Sleep Quality: Aiding in Restorative Rest

Quality sleep is essential for overall health and plays a role in diabetes management. Regular physical activity has been linked to improved sleep quality and duration.

- **Regulating Sleep Patterns:** Exercise can help regulate sleep patterns, contributing to better sleep quality. Establishing a consistent exercise routine may aid in falling asleep faster and experiencing deeper, more restorative sleep.

- **Managing Stress-Related Sleep Issues:** Since exercise is a stress-reducer, engaging in physical activity can help manage sleep issues related to stress or anxiety. Improved mental well-being positively influences sleep.

Reduced Risk of Complications: Long-Term Benefits

Consistent engagement in physical activity contributes to long-term benefits, reducing the risk of diabetes-related complications.

- **Prevention of Cardiovascular Complications:** By supporting cardiovascular health, exercise helps mitigate the risk of heart disease, stroke, and other cardiovascular complications associated with diabetes.

- **Improved Peripheral Circulation:** Regular physical activity enhances peripheral circulation, reducing the risk of complications such as peripheral artery disease and promoting overall vascular health.

- **Enhanced Nerve Function:** Exercise has been shown to positively impact nerve function, potentially reducing the risk of diabetic neuropathy—a condition characterized by nerve damage.

The benefits of exercise for diabetes control are vast and encompass improvements in blood sugar regulation, weight management, cardiovascular health, mood, mental well-being, sleep quality, and long-term complications. Incorporating regular physical activity into your routine empowers you to take an active role in managing your diabetes and promoting overall health.

Designing an Exercise Routine for Your Needs

Designing a personalized exercise routine that aligns with your needs and preferences is a crucial step toward incorporating regular physical activity into your lifestyle. Tailoring your exercise plan to your fitness level, health goals, and individual preferences enhances adherence and ensures a sustainable approach. Let's explore the key elements of designing an exercise routine for individuals with diabetes.

Assessing Your Fitness Level and Health Status

Before embarking on an exercise routine, it's essential to assess your current fitness level and health status. This assessment provides a foundation for designing a safe and effective exercise plan.

- **Consulting with Healthcare Providers:** Before starting a new exercise program, consult with your healthcare team, including your primary care physician and any specialists involved in your diabetes care. They can offer insights into any specific considerations or precautions based on your health status.

- **Fitness Assessment:** Consider undergoing a fitness assessment, which may include measurements of cardiovascular fitness, flexibility, strength, and balance. A fitness professional or physical therapist can assist in conducting these assessments.

- **Individualized Considerations:** Take into account any individual considerations, such as existing health conditions, joint issues, or complications related to diabetes. Designing an exercise routine that accommodates these factors ensures a safe and tailored approach.

Setting Realistic and Achievable Goals

Establishing clear and achievable goals is a key motivator and provides a roadmap for your exercise journey. Consider both short-term and long-term goals that align with your health and fitness aspirations.

- **Specificity of Goals:** Clearly define your goals, making them specific, measurable, achievable, relevant, and time-bound (SMART). For example, a goal might be to walk for 30 minutes most days of the week or to increase flexibility through regular stretching.

- **Gradual Progression:** Start with achievable goals and gradually progress over time. Avoid setting overly ambitious targets that may lead to burnout or injury. Incremental progress is sustainable and contributes to long-term success.

- **Diversification of Goals:** Consider diversifying your goals to include various aspects of fitness, such as cardiovascular endurance, strength, flexibility, and balance. A well-rounded approach contributes to overall health.

Choosing Enjoyable Activities: Enhancing Adherence

Selecting activities that you enjoy enhances adherence to your exercise routine. Engaging in activities that bring satisfaction and pleasure increases the likelihood of making exercise a consistent part of your lifestyle.

- **Identifying Preferences:** Consider your preferences when it comes to physical activities. Whether it's walking, cycling, swimming, dancing, or participating in group classes, choose activities that align with your interests.

- **Exploring Variety:** Keep your routine interesting by incorporating a variety of activities. This not only prevents monotony but also engages different muscle groups and promotes overall fitness.

- **Social Engagement:** If possible, consider activities that involve social engagement, such as group classes or exercising with a friend. Social support can contribute to motivation and enjoyment.

Incorporating Cardiovascular Exercise: A Foundation for Health

Cardiovascular exercise, also known as aerobic exercise, is foundational for heart health and overall fitness. Including cardiovascular activities in your routine supports blood sugar control, enhances endurance, and contributes to weight management.

- **Moderate-Intensity Activities:** Aim for at least 150 minutes of moderate-intensity aerobic exercise per week, spread across most days. This can include brisk walking, cycling, swimming, or other activities that elevate your heart rate.

- **Varying Intensity Levels:** Incorporate a mix of moderate and higher-intensity activities to challenge your cardiovascular system. Interval training, where you alternate between periods of higher and lower intensity, is one effective approach.

- **Enjoyable Cardiovascular Activities:** Choose cardiovascular activities that you find enjoyable. Whether it's dancing to your favorite music, participating in a fitness class, or hiking in nature, make it an activity you look forward to.

Integrating Strength Training: Supporting Muscle Health

Strength training, or resistance training, is essential for maintaining and building muscle mass. It contributes to improved metabolism, enhances strength, and supports overall physical function.

- **Frequency of Strength Training:** Include strength training exercises at least two days per week. Target major muscle groups, including the legs, hips, back, abdomen, chest, shoulders, and arms.

- **Using Resistance: Choose resistance levels that challenge your muscles without compromising form. Resistance can be provided by free weights, resistance bands, weight machines, or even your body weight.

- **Progressive Overload:** Gradually increase the intensity of your strength training routine by adjusting the resistance, number of repetitions, or sets. Progressive overload is key to ongoing improvements in strength.

Prioritizing Flexibility Exercises: Enhancing Range of Motion

Flexibility exercises, such as stretching, contribute to improved range of motion, joint health, and overall flexibility. Including stretching in your routine supports injury prevention and enhances functional mobility.

- **Dynamic and Static Stretching:** Incorporate both dynamic and static stretching into your routine. Dynamic stretches, such as leg swings and arm circles, are beneficial before exercise, while static stretches, such as holding a stretch position, are ideal for post-exercise flexibility.

- **Focus on Major Muscle Groups:** Target major muscle groups during your flexibility exercises. This includes stretches for the calves, thighs, hips, back, shoulders, and neck.

- **Regular Stretching Routine:** Dedicate time to stretching exercises on most days of the week. This routine can be incorporated into your warm-up and cool-down sessions or performed as a standalone activity.

Balancing with Stability and Balance Exercises

Stability and balance exercises are crucial, especially for individuals with diabetes who may be at an increased risk of falls or injuries. These exercises enhance core strength, improve stability, and contribute to overall body control.

- **Incorporating Core Exercises:** Include exercises that target the core muscles, such as planks, bridges, and abdominal exercises. A strong core supports posture, balance, and overall stability.

- **Balance Training:** Perform balance exercises to enhance proprioception and reduce the risk of falls. This can include activities such as standing on one leg, heel-to-toe walking, or using stability balls.

- **Proprioceptive Activities:** Engage in activities that improve proprioception, the body's awareness of its position in space. This can include activities like tai chi or yoga, which integrate balance and mindfulness.

Managing Blood Sugar During Physical Activity

Effectively managing blood sugar levels during physical activity is a crucial aspect of exercise for individuals with diabetes. Balancing insulin or medication dosages, monitoring blood sugar, and making informed decisions about nutrition and hydration contribute to a safe and successful exercise experience.

Pre-Exercise Preparations: Setting the Foundation

Preparing for physical activity involves considerations both before and during exercise to optimize blood sugar control.

- **Blood Sugar Monitoring:** Check your blood sugar levels before exercising, especially if you are taking insulin or certain medications. Monitoring provides valuable information about your starting point and helps guide adjustments.

- **Carbohydrate Intake:** Depending on your blood sugar levels, you may need to consume a small carbohydrate-containing snack before exercising. This can help prevent hypoglycemia (low blood sugar) during activity. The timing and amount of the snack will depend on individual needs.

- **Hydration:** Ensure adequate hydration before starting your exercise routine. Dehydration can affect blood volume and may impact blood sugar concentration.

Adjusting Insulin or Medication Dosages

For individuals using insulin or certain medications, adjusting dosages to accommodate the impact of exercise on blood sugar levels is crucial.

- **Consulting Healthcare Providers:** Work closely with your healthcare team, including your healthcare provider and diabetes educator, to determine appropriate adjustments to insulin or medication dosages.

- **Trial and Error:** Adjustments may require some trial and error. Factors such as the type, intensity, and duration of exercise, as well as individual responses, can influence the impact on blood sugar.

- **Understanding Insulin Sensitivity:** Recognize that insulin sensitivity may increase during and after exercise. This means that your body may require less insulin or medication to manage blood sugar effectively.

Hydration and Electrolyte Balance: Preventing Dehydration

Maintaining proper hydration and electrolyte balance is crucial for individuals with diabetes, especially during physical activity.

- **Hydration Guidelines:** Drink water before, during, and after exercise to prevent dehydration. The general recommendation is to consume about 8 ounces of water every 20 minutes during physical activity.

- **Monitoring Electrolytes:** Depending on the duration and intensity of exercise, electrolyte imbalances may occur. In cases of prolonged or intense activity, consider sports drinks that contain electrolytes. However, be mindful of the added sugars in these beverages.

Post-Exercise Considerations: Recovery and Monitoring

The period following exercise is equally important for blood sugar management and overall recovery.

- **Blood Sugar Monitoring Post-Exercise:** Check your blood sugar levels after exercising, especially if you've made adjustments to insulin or medication dosages. Monitoring helps you understand the impact of exercise on your blood sugar.

- **Post-Exercise Nutrition:** Consuming a balanced snack or meal after exercising supports recovery and helps stabilize blood sugar levels. Include a combination of carbohydrates, proteins, and healthy fats in your post-exercise nutrition.

- **Hydration for Recovery:** Continue to hydrate after exercise to support recovery. Water is typically sufficient for rehydration unless there has been significant fluid loss through sweat, in which case electrolyte-containing beverages may be beneficial.

Recognizing Hypoglycemia: Prompt Action and Prevention

Hypoglycemia, or low blood sugar, can occur during or after physical activity, especially if insulin or medication dosages are not adjusted appropriately.

- **Symptoms of Hypoglycemia:** Be aware of the signs of hypoglycemia, which can include shakiness, sweating, dizziness, confusion, and irritability. Prompt action is essential to address low blood sugar.

- **Carrying Rapid-Acting Carbohydrates:** Always have a source of rapid-acting carbohydrates on hand during exercise, such as glucose tablets, gels, or a small amount of juice. These can be used to raise blood sugar quickly if needed.

- **Regular Monitoring During Activity:** If engaging in prolonged or intense exercise, monitor your blood sugar levels regularly to catch any early signs of hypoglycemia.

Individualized Approach: Tailoring Strategies

It's crucial to recognize that the management of blood sugar during physical activity is highly individualized. What works for one person may not be suitable for another. Therefore, adopting a personalized approach based on your specific needs, responses, and preferences is key.

- **Regular Communication with the Healthcare Team:** Maintain open communication with your healthcare team regarding your exercise routine and blood sugar management. They can provide ongoing guidance and support.

- **Experimentation and Learning:** Understand that managing blood sugar during exercise may involve some experimentation and learning. Pay attention to how your body responds to different types and intensities of activity.

- **Flexibility in Strategies:** Be flexible in your approach and be willing to adjust strategies based on changing circumstances. Factors such as stress, illness, and changes in routine can influence blood sugar responses.

Effective blood sugar management during physical activity involves careful planning, monitoring, and adjustments to insulin or medication dosages. By taking a proactive and individualized approach, individuals with diabetes can enjoy the numerous benefits of exercise while maintaining optimal blood sugar control.

Incorporating regular physical activity into your lifestyle is a powerful tool for diabetes management. The benefits extend beyond blood sugar control to encompass cardiovascular health, weight management, mood enhancement, improved sleep, and long-term prevention of complications. By designing a personalized exercise routine, setting realistic goals, and managing blood sugar effectively, you can make exercise a sustainable and enjoyable part of your diabetes care journey.

CHAPTER 6

Medications and Insulin Therapy

Medications play a crucial role in the management of diabetes, providing individuals with effective tools to control blood sugar levels and reduce the risk of complications. In this chapter, we will explore the diverse landscape of diabetes medications, delve into the intricacies of insulin therapy and administration, and discuss strategies for navigating potential side effects and interactions associated with these treatments.

Overview of Diabetes Medications

The array of diabetes medications available today reflects the complexity of the condition and the need for tailored approaches to treatment. Understanding the different classes of medications, their mechanisms of action, and when they are prescribed is essential for individuals with diabetes and their healthcare providers.

Oral Medications: Targeting Various Pathways

Oral medications are a common first-line treatment for type 2 diabetes, aiming to improve insulin sensitivity, reduce glucose production by the liver, and enhance the effectiveness of insulin.

- **Metformin:** Often considered the first choice for type 2 diabetes, metformin works by reducing glucose production in the liver and improving insulin sensitivity in the muscles.

- **Sulfonylureas:** These medications stimulate the pancreas to release more insulin. Examples include glipizide, glyburide, and glimepiride.

- **Meglitinides:** Similar to sulfonylureas, meglitinides prompt the pancreas to release insulin, but their effect is shorter-lived. Repaglinide and nateglinide are examples.

- **Thiazolidinediones (TZDs):** TZDs improve insulin sensitivity in the muscles and adipose tissue. Examples include pioglitazone and rosiglitazone.

- **Dipeptidyl Peptidase-4 Inhibitors (DPP-4 Inhibitors):** These medications increase insulin release and decrease glucagon production. Sitagliptin, saxagliptin, and linagliptin are examples.

- **Sodium-Glucose Co-Transporter-2 Inhibitors (SGLT2 Inhibitors):** These drugs reduce glucose reabsorption in the kidneys, leading to increased glucose excretion in the urine. Canagliflozin, dapagliflozin, and empagliflozin belong to this class.

- **Alpha-Glucosidase Inhibitors:** These medications slow down the digestion of carbohydrates, helping to control post-meal blood sugar levels. Acarbose and miglitol are examples.

Injectable Medications: Enhancing Insulin Action

For individuals with type 2 diabetes who require more intensive treatment, injectable medications become a crucial component. These medications often work in conjunction with oral medications to provide comprehensive blood sugar control.

- **Glucagon-like Peptide-1 Receptor Agonists (GLP-1 RAs):** GLP-1 RAs stimulate the release of insulin and inhibit glucagon secretion. They also slow down gastric emptying, promoting a feeling of fullness. Examples include exenatide, liraglutide, and dulaglutide.

- **Amylin Analogs:** Pramlintide is an injectable medication that mimics the effects of amylin, a hormone that works alongside insulin to regulate blood sugar levels.

Understanding Insulin Therapy and Administration

Insulin therapy is a cornerstone in the management of diabetes, particularly for individuals with type 1 diabetes and some with type 2 diabetes who require more intensive blood sugar control. Understanding the different types of insulin, their onset and duration of action, and proper administration techniques is crucial for successful insulin therapy.

Types of Insulin: Tailoring to Individual Needs

Insulin is categorized based on its onset, peak, and duration of action. This categorization helps healthcare providers tailor insulin regimens to individual needs and lifestyle factors.

- **Rapid-Acting Insulin:** These insulins have a rapid onset and a short duration of action, making them ideal for mealtime bolus doses. Examples include insulin lispro, insulin aspart, and insulin glulisine.

- **Short-Acting Insulin:** Short-acting insulins have a slightly slower onset compared to rapid-acting insulins but are still used for mealtime bolus doses. Regular insulin is an example.

- **Intermediate-Acting Insulin:** This type of insulin has a more prolonged duration of action and is often used to cover basal insulin needs. NPH insulin is an example.

- **Long-Acting Insulin:** Long-acting insulins provide a steady release of insulin over an extended period, covering basal insulin needs. Examples include insulin glargine, insulin detemir, and insulin degludec.

- **Pre-Mixed Insulin:** These insulins combine a specific ratio of rapid-acting or short-acting insulin with intermediate-acting insulin. They are convenient for individuals who require both basal and bolus coverage.

Insulin Delivery Methods: From Syringes to Pumps

Various methods are available for administering insulin, allowing individuals to choose the approach that best fits their preferences and lifestyle.

- **Insulin Syringes:** Traditional insulin syringes are a common and cost-effective method of insulin delivery. They require individuals to draw the insulin from a vial before injection.

- **Insulin Pens:** Insulin pens are pre-filled devices that allow for convenient and accurate dosing. They are available in both disposable and reusable forms, providing a discreet and user-friendly option.

- **Insulin Pumps:** Insulin pumps are small devices that deliver a continuous supply of insulin throughout the day (basal rate) and allow for additional doses at mealtime (bolus doses). Pumps offer precise control and flexibility in insulin delivery.

- **Insulin Jet Injectors:** These devices use high-pressure air to deliver insulin through the skin, eliminating the need for needles. While less common, they provide an alternative for those averse to traditional injections.

Proper insulin administration involves more than just choosing the right type of insulin and delivery method. Technique plays a crucial role in ensuring accurate dosing and optimal blood sugar control.

- **Site Rotation:** Rotating injection sites helps prevent the development of lipodystrophy—a condition characterized by fatty tissue changes that can affect insulin absorption. Common injection sites include the abdomen, thighs, and buttocks.

- **Proper Storage:** Insulin should be stored according to the manufacturer's recommendations. Exposing insulin to extreme temperatures can affect its efficacy.

- **Injection Depth:** The depth of injection can influence insulin absorption. Subcutaneous injections are typically administered into the fatty tissue just beneath the skin.

- **Avoiding Air Bubbles:** Removing air bubbles from the insulin syringe or pen before injection ensures accurate dosing. Failing to do so may result in an incomplete dose.

- **Timing of Injections:** Administering insulin at the appropriate times, especially with mealtime doses, is crucial for effective blood sugar control. Rapid-acting insulins should be injected just before or shortly after meals.

Individualizing Insulin Regimens: Collaboration with Healthcare Providers

Achieving optimal blood sugar control with insulin therapy requires an individualized approach that considers factors such as lifestyle, activity level, dietary habits, and personal preferences.

- **Collaboration with Healthcare Providers:** Regular communication with healthcare providers is essential for adjusting insulin regimens based on changing needs. This collaboration allows for ongoing optimization of blood sugar management.

- **Self-Monitoring of Blood Sugar (SMBG):** Regular monitoring of blood sugar levels provides valuable information about how the body responds to insulin therapy. SMBG helps identify patterns and allows for timely adjustments.

- **Adjusting for Lifestyle Changes:** Changes in routine, physical activity or dietary habits may necessitate adjustments to insulin regimens. Working collaboratively with healthcare providers ensures that these changes are made thoughtfully.

- **Education and Empowerment:** Individuals on insulin therapy benefit from education on self-adjustment of insulin doses based on specific guidelines provided by healthcare providers. This empowerment fosters a sense of control over diabetes management.

Navigating Medication Side Effects and Interactions

While medications and insulin are essential tools in diabetes management, they may be accompanied by side effects and interactions that require attention. Being informed about potential issues and knowing how to navigate them is crucial for maintaining overall health.

Common Side Effects of Diabetes Medications: Understanding the Risks

Each class of diabetes medication comes with its own set of potential side effects. Understanding these risks allows individuals and healthcare providers to make informed decisions about treatment plans.

- **Hypoglycemia:** Many diabetes medications, particularly those that stimulate insulin release, carry the risk of hypoglycemia (low blood sugar). Recognizing symptoms such as shakiness, sweating, and dizziness is essential for prompt intervention.

- **Gastrointestinal Issues:** Some medications, especially metformin, may cause gastrointestinal side effects such as nausea, diarrhea, or abdominal discomfort. Taking medications with food or adjusting the dosage can sometimes alleviate these issues.

- **Weight Changes:** Certain medications, such as sulfonylureas and thiazolidinediones, may be associated with weight gain. Conversely, medications like GLP-1 RAs may contribute to weight loss.

- **Edema:** Thiazolidinediones, in particular, may lead to fluid retention and edema. Monitoring for signs of swelling and reporting them to healthcare providers is important.

- **Injection Site Reactions:** Individuals using injectable medications may experience redness, swelling, or irritation at the injection site. Rotating injection sites and proper technique can help minimize these reactions.

Interactions with Other Medications: Ensuring Compatibility

Individuals with diabetes often have other health conditions that may require additional medications. Understanding potential interactions between diabetes medications and other drugs is crucial to prevent adverse effects.

- **Communication with Healthcare Providers:** Informing healthcare providers about all medications, including over-the-counter drugs, supplements, and herbal remedies, is essential. This allows for a comprehensive assessment of potential interactions.

- **Adjustments in Medication Regimens:** Healthcare providers may need to make adjustments to diabetes medication regimens when introducing or modifying other medications. This ensures that blood sugar control is not compromised.

- **Monitoring for Adverse Effects:** Regular monitoring for adverse effects and symptoms of interactions is important. Changes in health or the onset of new symptoms should be promptly reported to healthcare providers.

- **Individualized Approaches:** Recognizing that medication interactions are highly individualized, healthcare providers tailor treatment plans based on the specific needs and health profile of each individual.

Strategies for Minimizing Side Effects: Enhancing Medication Tolerance

Minimizing side effects and optimizing medication tolerance involves a combination of lifestyle modifications, proper medication management, and ongoing communication with healthcare providers.

- **Gradual Introductions:** Introducing new medications gradually allows the body to adjust and minimizes the likelihood of severe side effects. This approach is particularly relevant when starting insulin therapy.

- **Dose Adjustments:** Modifying medication dosages under the guidance of healthcare providers can help balance the benefits of blood sugar control with the risk of side effects.

- **Monitoring and Reporting:** Regular monitoring of blood sugar levels, coupled with vigilance for potential side effects, empowers individuals to take an active role in their healthcare. Prompt reporting of concerns to healthcare providers ensures timely intervention.

- **Lifestyle Modifications:** Making lifestyle adjustments, such as changes in diet, exercise, and stress management, can complement medication therapy. These modifications may reduce the impact of certain side effects.

Navigating the landscape of diabetes medications and insulin therapy requires a comprehensive understanding of the available options, individualized treatment plans, and proactive management of potential side effects and interactions. By fostering open communication with healthcare providers, staying informed about treatment options, and actively participating in the decision-making process, individuals with diabetes can optimize their medication regimens for effective blood sugar control and overall well-being.

CHAPTER 7

Coping with Diabetes-Related Challenges

Living with diabetes presents a unique set of challenges, both physical and emotional. This chapter explores practical strategies for dealing with hypoglycemia (low blood sugar) and hyperglycemia (high blood sugar), managing stress and emotional well-being, and addressing diabetes burnout while staying motivated on your journey to a healthier life.

Dealing with Hypoglycemia (Low Blood Sugar) and Hyperglycemia (High Blood Sugar)

Balancing blood sugar levels is a delicate act for individuals with diabetes. Dealing with both hypoglycemia (low blood sugar) and hyperglycemia (high blood sugar) requires a nuanced approach that combines awareness, prevention, and prompt intervention.

Understanding Hypoglycemia: Recognizing and Responding

Hypoglycemia occurs when blood sugar levels drop below the normal range, leading to symptoms such as shakiness, sweating, irritability, and confusion. Managing hypoglycemia involves a multi-faceted approach.

- **Recognizing Early Signs:** Awareness of early signs of hypoglycemia is crucial for prompt intervention. Symptoms may vary among individuals but can include trembling, sweating, rapid heartbeat, and difficulty concentrating.

- **Prompt Glucose Intake:** In the event of hypoglycemia, consuming a fast-acting source of glucose is essential. This can include glucose tablets, gel, juice, or other high-sugar snacks. The goal is to raise blood sugar levels quickly and effectively.

- **Regular Monitoring:** Regular monitoring of blood sugar levels, especially around mealtime and before physical activity, helps identify patterns and prevent hypoglycemia. Adjusting medication dosages under the guidance of healthcare providers can further minimize the risk.

- **Carrying Emergency Supplies:** Individuals prone to hypoglycemia should always carry emergency supplies, such as glucose tablets or a small snack, to address low blood sugar levels promptly. Preparedness is key to managing unexpected situations.

Addressing Hyperglycemia: Strategies for Blood Sugar Control

Hyperglycemia, or high blood sugar, is a common concern for individuals with diabetes. Effective management involves a combination of lifestyle modifications, medication adherence, and regular monitoring.

- **Regular Blood Sugar Monitoring:** Monitoring blood sugar levels regularly provides insights into how various factors, including diet, exercise, and medication, impact glucose levels. Consistent monitoring allows for timely adjustments to prevent prolonged hyperglycemia.

- **Adhering to Medication Regimens:** Taking prescribed medications as directed by healthcare providers is fundamental to managing blood sugar levels. Skipping doses or adjusting medications without guidance can contribute to hyperglycemia.

- **Balanced Nutrition:** Adopting a balanced and carbohydrate-controlled diet is essential for blood sugar control. Working with a registered dietitian can help create personalized meal plans that align with individual health goals and preferences.

- **Regular Exercise:** Physical activity plays a key role in managing blood sugar levels. Regular exercise improves insulin sensitivity and helps regulate glucose levels. However, it's important to monitor blood sugar before, during, and after exercise to prevent fluctuations.

- **Hydration:** Staying well-hydrated supports overall health and can contribute to blood sugar control. Adequate hydration helps the kidneys function optimally, assisting in the removal of excess glucose from the bloodstream.

Managing Stress and Emotional Well-being

The emotional toll of living with diabetes is significant, and stress can exacerbate the challenges associated with managing the condition. Understanding how to manage stress and prioritize emotional well-being is integral to overall health.

Impact of Stress on Blood Sugar Levels: Making the Connection

Stress, whether physical or emotional, can impact blood sugar levels in various ways. Understanding this connection allows individuals with diabetes to implement strategies that mitigate stress-induced fluctuations.

- **Stress Hormones and Blood Sugar:** Stress triggers the release of hormones such as cortisol and adrenaline, which can elevate blood sugar levels. This physiological response is known as the "fight or flight" response.

- **Mind-Body Connection:** The mind-body connection plays a crucial role in diabetes management. Practices such as mindfulness, meditation, and deep breathing can help reduce stress and positively influence blood sugar control.

- **Identifying Stressors:** Recognizing specific stressors in daily life allows individuals to develop targeted strategies for managing stress. This may involve work-related stress, family dynamics, or lifestyle factors.

- **Holistic Approaches:** Adopting holistic approaches to stress management, such as yoga or tai chi, combines physical activity with relaxation techniques. These practices not only benefit stress levels but also contribute to overall well-being.

Strategies for Stress Management: Building Resilience

Effective stress management involves a combination of proactive strategies and coping mechanisms. Building resilience and incorporating stress-reducing activities into daily life can significantly impact emotional well-being.

- **Regular Physical Activity:** Engaging in regular physical activity is a powerful stress reducer. Exercise releases endorphins, improves mood, and provides an outlet for pent-up tension.

- **Mindfulness and Meditation:** Practices that promote mindfulness and meditation can help individuals become more aware of their thoughts and reactions to stress. Mindfulness-based stress reduction (MBSR) programs have shown efficacy in reducing stress in individuals with diabetes.

- **Setting Realistic Goals:** Setting achievable and realistic goals helps prevent feelings of overwhelm. Breaking down larger tasks into smaller, manageable steps fosters a sense of accomplishment and reduces stress.

- **Social Support:** Seeking support from friends, family, or diabetes support groups can provide an outlet for expressing feelings and sharing experiences. The emotional support of others is invaluable in navigating the challenges of diabetes.

- **Time Management:** Effectively managing time and prioritizing tasks can reduce stress associated with deadlines and competing responsibilities. Planning ahead and creating a structured routine contribute to a sense of control.

Handling Diabetes Burnout and Staying Motivated

Living with diabetes is a lifelong journey that may lead to periods of burnout—feeling overwhelmed, fatigued, and disengaged from diabetes management. Recognizing diabetes burnout and finding ways to stay motivated are essential for long-term well-being.

Recognizing Diabetes Burnout: Signs and Symptoms

Diabetes burnout is a state of emotional exhaustion and detachment from diabetes self-care tasks. Recognizing the signs and symptoms early allows individuals to address burnout proactively and seek support.

- **Feelings of Overwhelm:** Overwhelming feelings about managing diabetes tasks, such as monitoring blood sugar, taking medications, and adhering to dietary restrictions, may signal burnout.

- **Emotional Distress:** Increased emotional distress, including frustration, irritability, or feelings of failure, may be indicative of burnout. Emotional well-being is closely tied to diabetes management.

- **Avoidance of Diabetes Tasks:** Actively avoiding or neglecting diabetes-related tasks, such as skipping blood sugar checks or medication doses, may be a sign of burnout. This behavior can contribute to deteriorating health.

- **Changes in Lifestyle Habits:** Burnout may manifest as changes in lifestyle habits, including poor dietary choices, reduced physical activity, and disrupted sleep patterns. These changes can negatively impact blood sugar control.

Strategies for Coping with Diabetes Burnout: Regaining Momentum

Coping with diabetes burnout requires a combination of self-reflection, support from healthcare providers, and the implementation of strategies to regain motivation and momentum.

- **Open Communication with Healthcare Providers:** Sharing feelings of burnout with healthcare providers fosters a collaborative approach to managing diabetes. Providers can offer support, adjust treatment plans if necessary, and provide resources for additional assistance.

- **Setting Realistic Expectations:** Reevaluating and setting realistic expectations for diabetes management can help alleviate burnout. Acknowledging that perfection is not achievable and celebrating small victories are essential components of this mindset shift.

- **Seeking Emotional Support:** Seeking emotional support from friends, family, or mental health professionals can provide an outlet for expressing feelings of burnout. Support groups or therapy sessions offer a safe space to discuss challenges and find solutions.

- **Incorporating Variety into Diabetes Care:** Introducing variety into diabetes care routines can prevent monotony and enhance motivation. Trying new recipes, exploring different forms of exercise, or incorporating technology into blood sugar monitoring are examples of adding variety.

Staying Motivated for Long-Term Diabetes Management

Motivation is a key factor in sustaining long-term diabetes management. Cultivating a positive mindset, setting achievable goals, and celebrating successes contribute to ongoing motivation.

- **Goal Setting:** Setting specific, measurable, and achievable goals creates a roadmap for diabetes management. Break down larger goals into smaller, actionable steps to maintain motivation.

- **Tracking Progress:** Regularly tracking and celebrating progress reinforces a sense of accomplishment. Whether it's achieving target blood sugar levels, reaching a fitness milestone, or adhering to medication regimens, acknowledging success is important.

- **Incorporating Enjoyable Activities:** Incorporating enjoyable activities into diabetes care promotes adherence to self-care tasks. Whether it's trying new recipes, participating in a hobby, or engaging in physical activities you love, making diabetes care enjoyable is key.

- **Visualizing Long-Term Benefits:** Visualizing the long-term benefits of effective diabetes management, such as improved overall health, reduced risk of complications, and enhanced quality of life, motivates during challenging times.

Coping with diabetes-related challenges involves a holistic approach that encompasses physical and emotional well-being. By developing strategies to manage blood sugar fluctuations, implementing stress-reducing activities, recognizing and addressing burnout, and staying motivated for long-term care, individuals with diabetes can navigate their journey with resilience and a positive outlook. Regular collaboration with healthcare providers, seeking support from peers, and prioritizing self-care contribute to a balanced and fulfilling life with diabetes.

CHAPTER 8

Preventing and Managing Diabetes Complications

Living well with diabetes involves not only managing the day-to-day aspects of the condition but also addressing the potential long-term complications that can arise. This chapter explores the awareness and prevention of long-term complications, the importance of regular health check-ups and screenings, and strategies for managing diabetes-related complications effectively.

Long-Term Complications of Diabetes: Awareness and Prevention

Diabetes is a complex condition that, when not effectively managed, can lead to various long-term complications affecting different organ systems. Awareness of these complications and proactive prevention measures are key components of comprehensive diabetes care.

Cardiovascular Complications: Protecting Heart Health

Individuals with diabetes have an increased risk of cardiovascular complications, including heart disease and stroke. Understanding the factors contributing to these complications is crucial for prevention.

- **Blood Pressure Management:** High blood pressure is a common comorbidity in individuals with diabetes and is a major risk factor for cardiovascular complications. Regular monitoring and management of blood pressure through lifestyle modifications and medications when necessary are essential.

- **Cholesterol Control:** Diabetes can affect lipid levels, leading to an imbalance that increases the risk of atherosclerosis. Managing cholesterol levels through a heart-healthy diet, regular exercise, and medication if prescribed is important for preventing cardiovascular complications.

- **Blood Sugar Control:** Maintaining optimal blood sugar levels is fundamental in preventing cardiovascular complications. Consistent blood sugar monitoring, medication adherence, and lifestyle modifications contribute to overall heart health.

- **Lifestyle Modifications:** Adopting a heart-healthy lifestyle, including a balanced diet rich in fruits, vegetables, and whole grains, regular physical activity, and avoiding tobacco use, significantly contributes to the prevention of cardiovascular complications.

Neuropathy: Nurturing Nerve Health

Diabetic neuropathy is a condition characterized by nerve damage, often affecting the extremities. Preventive measures focus on maintaining nerve health and early intervention to mitigate symptoms.

- **Blood Sugar Control:** Consistent blood sugar control is crucial for preventing and slowing the progression of neuropathy. Elevated blood sugar levels contribute to nerve damage, emphasizing the importance of tight glycemic control.

- **Foot Care:** Regular foot care is essential for individuals with diabetes to prevent complications such as foot ulcers and infections. Daily inspection, proper hygiene, and wearing comfortable, well-fitted shoes are key aspects of foot care.

- **Regular Check-ups:** Periodic neurological examinations as part of routine healthcare check-ups help detect early signs of neuropathy. Early intervention can slow the progression of nerve damage.

- **Pain Management:** For those experiencing neuropathic pain, various medications and therapies can help manage symptoms. Consultation with healthcare providers is crucial to determine the most appropriate approach to pain management.

Nephropathy: Safeguarding Kidney Function

Diabetic nephropathy refers to kidney damage caused by diabetes. Protecting kidney function involves a combination of blood sugar control, blood pressure management, and regular monitoring.

- **Blood Sugar Control:** Tight glycemic control is paramount in preventing diabetic nephropathy. Monitoring blood sugar levels consistently and adhering to prescribed medications contribute to kidney health.

- **Blood Pressure Management:** Controlling blood pressure is equally important in safeguarding kidney function. Medications, if prescribed, lifestyle modifications, and regular check-ups help manage blood pressure effectively.

- **Proteinuria Monitoring:** Regular screening for proteinuria, an early sign of kidney damage, is essential for early detection and intervention. Timely measures can slow the progression of diabetic nephropathy.

- **Kidney-Friendly Diet:** Adopting a kidney-friendly diet that moderates protein intake, controls sodium, and emphasizes healthy foods support overall kidney health.

Retinopathy: Preserving Vision

Diabetic retinopathy is a complication affecting the eyes, potentially leading to vision impairment or blindness. Regular eye care and timely intervention are pivotal for preserving vision.

- **Regular Eye Exams:** Annual eye exams, including dilation of the pupils, help detect early signs of diabetic retinopathy. Early intervention, such as laser therapy or injections, can prevent vision loss.

- **Blood Sugar Control:** Maintaining consistent blood sugar levels is crucial for preventing and managing diabetic retinopathy. Elevated blood sugar contributes to damage in the small blood vessels of the retina.

- **Blood Pressure Management:** Controlling blood pressure is important for eye health. High blood pressure can exacerbate retinopathy, emphasizing the need for effective blood pressure management.

- **Lifestyle Modifications:** Healthy lifestyle habits, including a diet rich in antioxidants, regular exercise, and avoiding smoking, contribute to overall eye health.

Regular Health Check-ups and Screenings

Routine health check-ups and screenings are integral components of diabetes care. Regular monitoring helps identify potential complications early, allowing for timely intervention and management.

Comprehensive Physical Examinations: A Holistic Approach

Comprehensive physical examinations conducted by healthcare providers are crucial for assessing overall health and detecting potential complications associated with diabetes.

- **Blood Pressure Measurement:** Regular monitoring of blood pressure is essential for cardiovascular health. Elevated blood pressure is a common comorbidity in individuals with diabetes and requires timely management.

- **Neurological Examinations:** Periodic neurological examinations help detect early signs of neuropathy. Assessing reflexes, coordination, and sensation provides valuable insights into nerve health.

- **Foot Examinations:** Regular foot examinations are vital for preventing complications such as ulcers and infections. Healthcare providers assess skin integrity, circulation, and sensation during these examinations.

- **Eye Exams:** Annual eye exams, including dilation, are recommended to monitor for diabetic retinopathy and other eye-related complications. Early detection allows for timely intervention to preserve vision.

Dental Check-ups: Oral Health and Diabetes

Oral health is interconnected with diabetes, and individuals with diabetes are more prone to dental issues. Regular dental check-ups contribute to overall well-being.

- **Periodontal Examinations:** Periodontal examinations help identify early signs of gum disease, a condition more prevalent in individuals with diabetes. Timely dental care and good oral hygiene practices are essential.

- **Oral Hygiene Education:** Dental check-ups provide an opportunity for education on proper oral hygiene practices. Good oral hygiene is crucial for preventing gum disease and maintaining overall health.

- **Management of Dental Issues:** Prompt management of dental issues, such as cavities or gum disease, is important to prevent complications. Collaboration between healthcare providers and dentists ensures comprehensive care.

Blood Tests and Monitoring: Assessing Metabolic Control

Regular blood tests are fundamental for assessing metabolic control and detecting potential changes in blood sugar levels, lipid profiles, and kidney function.

- **Hemoglobin A1c Testing:** Hemoglobin A1c tests provide a comprehensive view of average blood sugar levels over the past few months. This test is crucial for assessing long-term glycemic control.

- **Lipid Profile Checks:** Monitoring lipid profiles helps assess cardiovascular risk. Lipid imbalances can contribute to atherosclerosis, emphasizing the importance of regular checks.

- **Kidney Function Tests:** Periodic kidney function tests, including serum creatinine and urine albumin-to-creatinine ratio, help assess renal health. Early detection of changes allows for timely intervention.

- **Liver Function Tests:** Liver function tests provide insights into liver health, which can be influenced by factors such as diabetes medications. Monitoring liver function is important for overall well-being.

Strategies for Managing Diabetes-Related Complications

Effective management of diabetes-related complications involves a combination of medical interventions, lifestyle modifications, and proactive strategies to address specific complications.

Cardiovascular Complications: Lifestyle and Medication Management

Cardiovascular complications necessitate a multifaceted approach involving lifestyle modifications and, in some cases, medications to manage risk factors.

- **Medication Adherence:** Adhering to prescribed medications for blood pressure and cholesterol management is crucial. Regular check-ups with healthcare providers allow for adjustments in medications as needed.

- **Heart-Healthy Diet:** Adopting a heart-healthy diet that prioritizes fruits, vegetables, whole grains, and lean proteins supports cardiovascular health. Reducing sodium intake and avoiding trans fats are additional dietary considerations.

- **Regular Exercise:** Physical activity contributes to cardiovascular health. Regular exercise helps control blood pressure, improve lipid profiles, and enhance overall well-being.

- **Smoking Cessation:** Smoking is a significant risk factor for cardiovascular complications. Quitting smoking is a critical step in managing and preventing heart-related issues.

Neuropathy: Symptomatic Management and Lifestyle Adaptations

Managing neuropathy involves addressing symptoms and making lifestyle adaptations to prevent further nerve damage.

- **Medication for Pain Management:** Medications for pain management, such as certain antidepressants or anticonvulsants, may be prescribed to alleviate neuropathic pain.

- **Foot Care Practices:** Regular foot care practices, including daily inspection, proper hygiene, and wearing comfortable shoes, are vital for preventing complications associated with neuropathy.

- **Physical Therapy:** Physical therapy may be recommended to improve strength, balance, and coordination, reducing the risk of falls and injuries.

Nephropathy: Blood Sugar and Blood Pressure Control

Effectively managing diabetic nephropathy involves tight control of blood sugar levels and blood pressure, as well as lifestyle modifications.

- **Blood Sugar Control:** Maintaining optimal blood sugar levels is crucial for preventing further kidney damage. Adhering to prescribed medications, dietary modifications, and regular monitoring contribute to glycemic control.

- **Blood Pressure Management:** Controlling blood pressure is equally important in managing nephropathy. Medications, lifestyle modifications, and regular check-ups help maintain blood pressure within target ranges.

- **Kidney-Friendly Diet:** Adopting a kidney-friendly diet, which may involve limiting protein intake and moderating sodium, supports overall kidney health.

Retinopathy: Ophthalmologic Interventions and Lifestyle Measures

Management of diabetic retinopathy involves ophthalmologic interventions, lifestyle measures, and regular eye care.

- **Ophthalmologic Interventions:** Laser therapy or injections may be recommended to address retinopathy and prevent further vision loss. Early intervention is crucial for optimal outcomes.

- **Blood Sugar Control:** Consistent blood sugar control is fundamental in managing and preventing retinopathy. Regular monitoring and adherence to prescribed medications contribute to glycemic control.

- **Eye-Protective Measures:** Wearing sunglasses and avoiding prolonged exposure to bright sunlight contribute to eye protection. These measures can help prevent worsening of retinopathy.

Preventing and managing diabetes complications requires a proactive and comprehensive approach. Awareness of potential long-term complications, regular health check-ups, and timely interventions contribute to overall well-being.

Strategies for managing specific complications involve a combination of medical treatments, lifestyle modifications, and ongoing collaboration with healthcare providers. By embracing a holistic approach to diabetes care, individuals can navigate their journey with resilience, minimize the impact of complications, and enhance their quality of life.

Regular communication with healthcare providers, adherence to prescribed treatments, and a commitment to a healthy lifestyle are key components of successful diabetes management.

CHAPTER 9

Support Systems and Lifestyle Adjustments

Living well with diabetes goes beyond individual management—it involves building a strong support network, effective communication with loved ones about your diabetes, and making lifestyle adjustments that allow you to thrive while managing your condition. This chapter explores the importance of building a support network with friends, family, and diabetes support groups, providing insights into communicating about your diabetes with loved ones, and offering guidance on navigating various aspects of life, including travel, socializing, pursuing hobbies and interests, all while maintaining a positive and fulfilling life with diabetes.

Building a Support Network: Friends, Family, and Diabetes Support Groups

The journey of living with diabetes does not need to be traveled alone. Building a robust support network is crucial for emotional well-being, encouragement, and practical assistance in managing the challenges that diabetes may bring.

Friends and Family: The Pillars of Support

Friends and family form the primary foundation of your support network. Their understanding, encouragement, and willingness to be part of your journey can make a significant impact on your ability to cope with diabetes.

- **Educating Your Inner Circle:** Start by providing your friends and family with information about diabetes. Help them understand the basics of the condition, its management, and how they can support you effectively.

Clear communication is key to fostering a supportive environment.

- **Encouraging Involvement:** Invite your loved ones to actively participate in your diabetes management. This could include attending medical appointments, learning about healthy eating habits, or even joining you in physical activities. Shared experiences strengthen bonds and create a sense of unity.

- **Emotional Support:** Living with a chronic condition like diabetes can be emotionally challenging. Friends and family can offer a listening ear, provide empathy, and offer words of encouragement. Their emotional support is invaluable in navigating the highs and lows of diabetes management.

- **Creating Inclusive Lifestyle Adjustments:** Incorporate your loved ones into lifestyle adjustments. Whether it's modifying family meals to align with your dietary needs or involving them in regular physical activities, making these adjustments together fosters a sense of shared responsibility.

Diabetes Support Groups: Connecting with Peers

Beyond friends and family, diabetes support groups offer a unique space to connect with individuals who share similar experiences. Joining these groups provides a sense of community, shared knowledge, and a platform to discuss challenges and successes.

- **Local Support Groups:** Many communities have local diabetes support groups that meet regularly. These groups often provide a safe space for individuals to share their experiences, ask questions, and learn from one another. Local resources and insights can be particularly valuable.

- **Online Communities:** In the digital age, online diabetes communities and forums offer a convenient way to connect with a broader audience. These platforms provide a wealth of information, allowing you to tap into the collective wisdom of individuals from different backgrounds and experiences.

- **Attending Workshops and Events:** Diabetes-related workshops and events are excellent opportunities to connect with peers. Whether in-person or virtual, these gatherings often feature expert speakers, interactive sessions, and the chance to build lasting connections with others in the diabetes community.

- **Seeking Professional Guidance:** Healthcare providers can also guide you to reputable support groups or educational programs. They may have information on local resources or recommend online platforms that align with your preferences and needs.

Communicating with Loved Ones about Your Diabetes

Effective communication about your diabetes with loved ones is essential for garnering support, fostering understanding, and creating an environment conducive to your well-being. Clear and open communication ensures that your needs are met and that your loved ones can actively participate in your care.

Choosing the Right Time and Setting

Initiating a conversation about diabetes requires thoughtful consideration of the timing and setting. Choose a calm and private environment where everyone can focus on the discussion without distractions.

- **Timing Matters:** Select a time when all parties involved are relaxed and not preoccupied with other pressing matters. Avoid bringing up the topic during stressful moments or when emotions are running high.

- **Create a Comfortable Setting:** Choose a comfortable setting that promotes open communication. This could be at home, during a walk, or in a quiet space where everyone feels at ease.

- **Setting the Tone:** Begin the conversation with a positive and constructive tone. Emphasize the collaborative nature of diabetes management and express the importance of having everyone on the same page.

Educating Your Loved Ones

Education is a crucial component of effective communication. Providing your loved ones with accurate information about diabetes helps dispel myths, reduces stigma, and fosters a better understanding of your needs.

- **Share Basic Information:** Start by sharing basic information about diabetes, including its types, causes, and daily management. Use simple language to ensure that everyone can grasp the fundamental concepts.

- **Discuss Your Specific Type of Diabetes:** If you have a specific type of diabetes, such as type 1 or type 2, explain the nuances of your condition. Clarify any misconceptions and outline how your management may differ from what they might have heard or assumed.

- **Highlight the Importance of Support:** Emphasize that your well-being is significantly influenced by the support you receive. Discuss how their understanding and involvement can positively impact your ability to manage diabetes effectively.

- **Address Emotional Aspects:** Acknowledge the emotional aspects of living with diabetes. Share your feelings, concerns, and any challenges you may face. Encourage open dialogue about how everyone can contribute to a supportive emotional environment.

Practical Involvement and Lifestyle Adjustments

Once your loved ones have a foundational understanding of diabetes, involve them in practical aspects of your care and lifestyle adjustments. This can include meal planning, physical activities, and support during medical appointments.

- **Meal Planning Together:** Involve your loved ones in meal planning, grocery shopping, and cooking. This not only makes them active participants in your care but also fosters a sense of unity in making healthier food choices.

- **Participating in Physical Activities:** Engage in physical activities together, whether it's daily walks, workout sessions, or other forms of exercise. Physical activity benefits everyone and reinforces the importance of an active lifestyle in diabetes management.

- **Accompanying to Medical Appointments:** Invite a trusted family member or friend to accompany you to medical appointments. This provides them with firsthand knowledge of your care plan and allows healthcare providers to address any questions or concerns they may have.

- **Creating a Supportive Environment:** Work together to create a supportive environment at home. This may involve organizing diabetes-friendly snacks, ensuring a well-stocked supply of medications, or establishing a routine that accommodates your diabetes management needs.

Traveling, Socializing, Pursuing Hobbies and Interests, and Living Well with Diabetes

Managing diabetes should not restrict your ability to travel, socialize, or pursue hobbies and interests. With thoughtful planning and an understanding support system, you can lead a fulfilling life while effectively managing your condition.

Traveling with Diabetes: Preparation and Adaptation

Traveling can present unique challenges for individuals with diabetes, but with careful planning and preparation, you can enjoy your journeys while effectively managing your health.

- **Pre-Trip Planning:** Plan your trip well in advance, considering factors such as time zone changes, meal schedules, and physical activity. Consult with your healthcare provider to discuss any adjustments to your medication or insulin regimen.

- **Carrying Essential Supplies:** Ensure that you have an adequate supply of medications, testing supplies, and snacks. Pack them in your carry-on bag to have easy access during the journey. Consider carrying a medical alert card or bracelet indicating that you have diabetes.

- **Adapting to Local Cuisine:** Research the local cuisine at your destination and plan your meals accordingly. Familiarize yourself with the carbohydrate content of common dishes, and be prepared to make adjustments to your insulin or medication doses.

- **Staying Hydrated:** Traveling can be dehydrating, so it's important to stay well-hydrated. Carry a reusable water bottle and make a conscious effort to drink water regularly, especially if you're flying.

Socializing and Dining Out: Making Informed Choices

Socializing and dining out are integral parts of life, and having diabetes shouldn't hinder your ability to enjoy these activities. With mindful choices and open communication, you can navigate social situations successfully.

- **Communicating Dietary Preferences:** When invited to social events or restaurants, don't hesitate to communicate your dietary preferences or restrictions. Most hosts and establishments are accommodating and willing to make adjustments to meet your needs.

- **Making Smart Food Choices:** When dining out, opt for healthier menu choices, such as grilled proteins, vegetables, and whole grains. Be mindful of portion sizes and consider sharing dishes to manage carbohydrate intake.

- **Balancing Alcohol Consumption:** If you choose to consume alcohol, do so in moderation and be aware of its potential impact on blood sugar levels. Monitor your blood sugar regularly, and consider having a snack along with your drink.

- **Planning for Special Occasions:** For special occasions, plan ahead by adjusting your medication or insulin doses as needed. Communicate your plans with your healthcare provider to receive guidance on managing your diabetes during events or celebrations.

Pursuing Hobbies and Interests: Integrating Diabetes Care

Diabetes management can seamlessly integrate into your hobbies and interests. Whether you enjoy sports, arts, or other activities, there are ways to align your passions with your health needs.

- **Physical Activities:** Engage in physical activities that align with your interests, whether it's hiking, swimming, or dancing. Regular exercise not only supports diabetes management but also contributes to overall well-being.

- **Artistic Pursuits:** If you have artistic hobbies, such as painting, writing, or playing a musical instrument, use these creative outlets as a form of stress relief. Expressing yourself through art can positively impact your emotional health.

- **Joining Diabetes-Focused Groups:** Explore diabetes-focused clubs or groups that align with your hobbies. Whether it's a diabetes-friendly cooking class, a walking group, or an art therapy session, connecting with like-minded individuals can be both enjoyable and supportive.

- **Incorporating Physical Activity into Hobbies:** Find ways to incorporate physical activity into your hobbies. For example, if you enjoy gardening, consider the physical benefits of tending to your garden. This dual approach enhances both your hobby and your health.

Living Well with Diabetes: A Holistic Approach

Living well with diabetes is about adopting a holistic approach that encompasses physical, emotional, and social well-being. Balancing these aspects of life ensures a fulfilling and positive journey with diabetes.

- **Prioritizing Self-Care:** Prioritize self-care by dedicating time to activities that bring joy and relaxation. This could include reading, meditation, or spending time in nature. Self-care contributes to emotional well-being and resilience in diabetes management.

- **Regular Health Check-ups:** Stay proactive in managing your health by attending regular health check-ups. These appointments allow healthcare providers to monitor your diabetes, address any concerns, and make adjustments to your care plan.

- **Celebrating Achievements:** Acknowledge and celebrate your achievements, whether they are related to blood sugar control, lifestyle changes, or personal milestones. Recognizing your successes contributes to a positive mindset.

- **Maintaining a Positive Mindset:** Cultivate a positive mindset by focusing on the aspects of life you can control. While diabetes may present challenges, maintaining a hopeful and optimistic outlook contributes to overall well-being.

- **Seeking Professional Support:** If you encounter challenges or emotional struggles, don't hesitate to seek professional support. Mental health professionals can provide guidance, coping strategies, and a safe space to discuss the emotional aspects of living with diabetes.

Support systems and lifestyle adjustments play a pivotal role in the journey of living well with diabetes. Building a strong support network with friends, family, and fellow individuals with diabetes creates a foundation of understanding and encouragement. Effective communication with loved ones fosters a supportive environment, ensuring that your needs are met while making lifestyle adjustments. Navigating various aspects of life, including travel, socializing, pursuing hobbies, and living well with diabetes, requires a proactive and positive mindset. With the right support, communication, and lifestyle adjustments, individuals can embrace a fulfilling and active life while effectively managing their diabetes.

Regular collaboration with healthcare providers, staying informed about diabetes management, and maintaining a balance between physical and emotional well-being contribute to a holistic and thriving life with diabetes.

CHAPTER 10

Thriving with Diabetes: Tips for a Fulfilling Life

Living with diabetes doesn't just mean managing the condition—it's about thriving, finding fulfillment, and leading a life rich in experiences. This chapter explores essential tips for thriving with diabetes, including setting realistic goals and celebrating successes, embracing self-care and prioritizing well-being, and finding inspiration and motivation on your diabetes journey.

Setting Realistic Goals and Celebrating Successes

Setting and achieving realistic goals is a powerful tool for managing diabetes effectively. Goals provide direction, motivation, and a sense of accomplishment. Here's how to set realistic goals and celebrate the successes along the way.

Understanding the Importance of Goals

Goals serve as a roadmap for your diabetes management, helping you stay focused and motivated. Whether they are related to blood sugar control, lifestyle changes, or overall well-being, setting goals provides a sense of purpose and direction.

- **Long-Term and Short-Term Goals:** Differentiate between long-term and short-term goals. Long-term goals might include achieving a target A1c level or losing a certain amount of weight. Short-term goals could be daily or weekly targets that contribute to the larger objectives.

- **Health and Lifestyle Goals:** Goals related to health outcomes, such as maintaining target blood sugar levels, managing cholesterol, or achieving a healthy weight, are essential. Additionally, lifestyle goals, such as incorporating regular physical activity or adopting a balanced diet, contribute to overall well-being.

- **Emotional and Psychological Goals:** Consider goals related to emotional and psychological well-being. This could involve managing stress, practicing mindfulness, or seeking professional support for emotional health. A holistic approach to goal-setting addresses both physical and emotional aspects of diabetes management.

Setting SMART Goals

The SMART criteria (Specific, Measurable, Achievable, Relevant, Time-bound) provide a framework for setting effective and achievable goals.

- **Specific:** Clearly define your goal. Instead of a vague goal like "improve blood sugar control," specify "maintain fasting blood sugar levels below 120 mg/dL consistently."

- **Measurable:** Set criteria to measure progress. For example, if the goal is increased physical activity, specify the number of minutes or steps per day.

- **Achievable:** Ensure that the goal is realistic and attainable. Consider your current lifestyle, commitments, and capabilities when setting goals.

- **Relevant:** Align the goal with your overall diabetes management plan. If weight loss is a goal, ensure it aligns with your healthcare provider's recommendations.

- **Time-bound:** Set a timeframe for achieving the goal. This provides a sense of urgency and helps monitor progress. For instance, "achieve a 5% weight loss in three months."

Breaking Down Goals into Actionable Steps

Breaking larger goals into smaller, actionable steps makes them more manageable and increases the likelihood of success.

- **Identify Steps Toward the Goal:** List specific actions you need to take to achieve the goal. For example, if the goal is to increase vegetable intake, actionable steps could include planning meals with more vegetables or trying a new vegetable each week.

- **Create a Schedule:** Incorporate goal-related activities into your daily or weekly schedule. Consistency is key to building habits that support your goals.

- **Monitor Progress:** Regularly assess your progress toward the goal. This could involve keeping a journal, using a tracking app, or discussing progress with your healthcare provider.

- **Adjust as Needed:** Be flexible and open to adjusting goals based on your experiences and feedback from healthcare providers. If a particular approach isn't working, consider modifying the goal or the steps toward achieving it.

Celebrating Successes

Celebrating successes, no matter how small, is vital for maintaining motivation and a positive mindset on your diabetes journey.

- **Acknowledge Achievements:** Take time to acknowledge and celebrate both big and small achievements. Whether it's reaching a weight loss milestone, consistently hitting blood sugar targets, or adopting a new healthy habit, recognition is crucial.

- **Reward Yourself:** Consider incorporating rewards into your goal-setting process. Treat yourself to something enjoyable when you achieve a milestone. This could be a relaxing day, a favorite meal, or a small purchase that brings joy.

- **Share Successes with Support System:** Share your successes with your support system—friends, family, or fellow individuals with diabetes. Celebrating together enhances the sense of accomplishment and strengthens your support network.

- **Reflect on Progress:** Regularly reflect on your progress and the positive changes you've made. This reflection reinforces your commitment and motivation to continue thriving with diabetes.

Embracing Self-Care and Prioritizing Your Well-being

Self-care is a fundamental aspect of thriving with diabetes. Prioritizing your well-being involves nurturing both your physical and emotional health. Here's how to embrace self-care as an integral part of your diabetes management.

Understanding the Importance of Self-Care

Self-care is not a luxury; it's a necessity, especially when managing a chronic condition like diabetes. Prioritizing your well-being contributes to better physical health, emotional resilience, and an overall improved quality of life.

- **Balancing Physical and Emotional Health:** Self-care involves maintaining a balance between physical and emotional health. While physical self-care includes aspects like medication adherence and regular exercise, emotional self-care encompasses stress management, mindfulness, and seeking emotional support.

- **Preventing Burnout:** Diabetes management can be demanding, and self-care plays a crucial role in preventing burnout. Taking breaks, practicing relaxation techniques, and incorporating enjoyable activities into your routine are essential for long-term well-being.

- **Enhancing Quality of Life:** Self-care enhances your overall quality of life. By prioritizing activities that bring joy, relaxation, and fulfillment, you contribute to a positive mindset and improved resilience in the face of diabetes-related challenges.

Incorporating Physical Self-Care Practices

Physical self-care practices are integral to diabetes management and overall well-being.

- **Regular Physical Activity:** Engage in regular physical activity that aligns with your preferences and health conditions. This could include walking, cycling, swimming, or other forms of exercise. Physical activity not only supports blood sugar control but also contributes to cardiovascular health and overall fitness.

- **Balanced Nutrition:** Adopting a balanced and diabetes-friendly diet is a key aspect of physical self-care. Work with a healthcare provider or a registered dietitian to create a meal plan that meets your nutritional needs and aligns with your diabetes management goals.

- **Adequate Sleep:** Prioritize getting adequate and quality sleep. Poor sleep can impact blood sugar levels and overall well-being. Establish a bedtime routine, create a comfortable sleep environment, and aim for consistent sleep patterns.

- **Regular Health Check-ups:** Schedule and attend regular health check-ups as recommended by your healthcare provider. These check-ups allow for the monitoring of your diabetes management, early detection of potential issues, and adjustments to your care plan as needed.

Prioritizing Emotional Self-Care Practices

Emotional self-care is equally important for thriving with diabetes.

- **Stress Management Techniques:** Practice stress management techniques such as deep breathing, meditation, or mindfulness. Chronic stress can negatively impact blood sugar levels, making stress reduction a valuable aspect of diabetes care.

- **Seeking Emotional Support:** Establish a support system for emotional well-being. Whether it's friends, family, or mental health professionals, having individuals you can turn to for emotional support is crucial. Joining diabetes support groups can also provide a unique platform for shared experiences and insights.

- **Setting Boundaries:** Establish and communicate clear boundaries to protect your emotional well-being. This could involve setting limits on work commitments, prioritizing personal time, and being mindful of stressors that may affect your emotional health.

- **Engaging in Enjoyable Activities:** Incorporate activities you enjoy into your routine. Whether it's reading, listening to music, or pursuing a hobby, allocating time for enjoyable activities contributes positively to your emotional well-being.

Creating a Holistic Self-Care Plan

A holistic self-care plan integrates both physical and emotional self-care practices into your daily life.

- **Assessing Individual Needs:** Identify your individual needs for physical and emotional well-being. Consider factors such as lifestyle, preferences, and any specific challenges related to diabetes management.

- **Customizing Self-Care Practices:** Tailor self-care practices to align with your preferences and lifestyle. The more personalized and enjoyable the self-care activities, the more likely you are to integrate them consistently into your routine.

- **Regularly Reviewing and Adapting:** Periodically review your self-care plan to ensure it remains effective and relevant. Life circumstances, goals, and priorities may change, requiring adjustments to your self-care practices.

- **Incorporating Variety:** Introduce variety into your self-care routine to prevent monotony. Trying new activities, exploring different forms of exercise, or incorporating diverse relaxation techniques adds richness to your self-care plan.

Maintaining inspiration and motivation is vital for long-term success in managing diabetes. Whether you're newly diagnosed or have been living with diabetes for years, finding sources of inspiration and staying motivated are ongoing processes.

Identifying Personal Motivators

Understanding what motivates you personally is the first step toward maintaining motivation in your diabetes journey.

- **Reflecting on Values and Goals:** Consider your core values and long-term goals. Connecting your diabetes management to these values and goals provides a deeper sense of purpose and motivation.

- **Acknowledging Achievements:** Regularly acknowledge and celebrate your achievements. Reflecting on the progress you've made, no matter how small, reinforces a positive mindset and motivates you to continue making positive choices.

- **Visualizing Long-Term Benefits:** Visualize the long-term benefits of effective diabetes management. Whether it's preventing complications, improving overall health, or enhancing your quality of life, keeping these outcomes in mind can be motivating.

- **Learning from Setbacks:** Instead of viewing setbacks as failures, consider them as opportunities for learning and growth. Analyze what contributed to the setback, adjust your approach, and use the experience to strengthen your commitment to diabetes management.

External sources of inspiration can provide ongoing encouragement and motivation.

- **Connecting with Peers:** Engage with individuals who share similar experiences. This could involve joining diabetes support groups, participating in online forums, or attending diabetes-related events. Shared stories and insights can be inspiring and offer valuable perspectives.

- **Exploring Success Stories:** Read or listen to success stories of individuals who have effectively managed diabetes. Learning about real-life experiences and achievements can instill a sense of hope and inspiration.

- **Educational Resources:** Stay informed about the latest developments in diabetes management. Educational resources, such as books, articles, and reputable websites, provide valuable information that can inspire proactive and informed choices.

- **Utilizing Technology:** Leverage technology to stay connected and motivated. Diabetes management apps, wearable devices, and online communities offer tools and platforms that facilitate tracking progress, setting goals, and receiving support.

Creating a Motivational Environment

Your physical and social environment can significantly impact your motivation.

- **Surrounding Yourself with Positivity:** Foster a positive and supportive environment. Surround yourself with individuals who uplift and encourage you. Limit exposure to negativity and seek out sources of positivity in your daily life.

- **Displaying Visual Reminders:** Create visual reminders of your goals and motivations. This could include a vision board, positive affirmations, or images that represent your aspirations. Place these reminders in prominent locations to reinforce your commitment.

- **Setting Regular Milestones:** Break down long-term goals into smaller milestones. Celebrating these milestones regularly provides a sense of achievement and maintains a positive momentum in your diabetes journey.

- **Engaging in Continuous Learning:** Stay curious and engaged in continuous learning about diabetes. This ongoing exploration can fuel your motivation by introducing new insights, strategies, and perspectives.

Thriving with diabetes is not only about effective management but also about cultivating a fulfilling life. Setting realistic goals and celebrating successes provide direction and motivation while embracing self-care ensures both physical and emotional well-being. Finding inspiration and staying motivated on your diabetes journey involves understanding personal motivators, seeking external sources of inspiration, and creating a motivational environment. Whether you're navigating the initial stages of a diabetes diagnosis or have been managing the condition for years, these tips contribute to a holistic and positive approach to living well with diabetes. By incorporating these practices into your daily life, you can not only manage diabetes effectively but also thrive, finding joy, purpose, and fulfillment in your journey.

Remember, each step forward is a victory, and embracing a positive mindset is a powerful tool in the ongoing adventure of thriving with diabetes.

CONCLUSION

Embracing Your New Life with Diabetes

Embarking on the journey of living with diabetes may feel like navigating uncharted waters. It's a journey that begins with the diagnosis, encompasses lifestyle adjustments, and unfolds as a continuous exploration of self-care, resilience, and empowerment. As you stand at this crossroads, it's essential to recognize that your new life with diabetes is not a limitation but an opportunity—an opportunity to take charge of your health, cultivate a positive mindset, and embrace a fulfilling life despite the challenges.

Reflecting on Your Journey

In this book, we've delved into the multifaceted aspects of living well with diabetes for the newly diagnosed. From understanding the different types, causes, and symptoms of diabetes to exploring the intricacies of diagnosis, initial steps, blood sugar monitoring, healthy eating, physical activity, medication, coping strategies, and preventing complications, each chapter has been a step on your journey toward empowerment and informed decision-making.

As you reflect on the chapters and the knowledge gained, it's important to acknowledge the resilience you've demonstrated. The process of understanding and managing diabetes is not a linear path; it's a dynamic and evolving journey. Your commitment to learning, adapting, and incorporating positive changes into your life is commendable.

Embracing a Holistic Approach

Living well with diabetes extends beyond managing blood sugar levels. It's about adopting a holistic approach that considers your physical health, emotional well-being, and the social aspects of your life. The chapters have guided you in setting realistic goals, celebrating successes, embracing self-care, finding motivation, and building a support network. These elements collectively contribute to a well-rounded and fulfilling life with diabetes.

Setting Realistic Goals and Celebrating Successes:

Setting realistic and achievable goals is a cornerstone of effective diabetes management. It's not about perfection but progress. By breaking down larger goals into manageable steps, you've created a roadmap for success. Whether it's maintaining target blood sugar levels, adopting healthier eating habits, or incorporating regular physical activity, every step forward is a triumph. Celebrating these successes, no matter how small, reinforces a positive mindset and fuels motivation for the journey ahead.

Embracing Self-Care and Prioritizing Your Well-being:

Self-care is not a luxury; it's a fundamental aspect of thriving with diabetes. The chapters have emphasized the importance of balancing physical and emotional self-care practices. Regular physical activity, balanced nutrition, adequate sleep, and regular health check-ups contribute to your physical well-being. At the same time, stress management, seeking emotional support, and engaging in enjoyable activities nurture your emotional health. By prioritizing self-care, you're investing in the foundation of a resilient and fulfilling life.

Finding Inspiration and Motivation on Your Diabetes Journey:

Maintaining inspiration and motivation is an ongoing process. By identifying personal motivators, connecting with peers, exploring success stories, and creating a motivational environment, you've cultivated a mindset that transcends the challenges of diabetes. Your ability to learn from setbacks, visualize long-term benefits, and stay curious about diabetes management reflects a proactive approach to your well-being.

Embracing Change with Resilience

Change is a constant companion in the journey with diabetes. From adjusting to a new dietary routine to incorporating physical activity into your daily life, adapting to change requires resilience. It's not about avoiding challenges but facing them with courage and a willingness to learn. Resilience is the cornerstone of your ability to navigate the twists and turns of your diabetes journey. It's the assurance that setbacks are not roadblocks but detours leading to newfound insights and strengths.

As you embrace change with resilience, remember that your journey is unique. What works for one person may not work the same way for another. The beauty of your uniqueness lies in the flexibility to tailor strategies, learn from experiences, and discover the approaches that best suit your individual needs.

Building and Nurturing Your Support System

A robust support system is a pillar of strength in your journey with diabetes. Whether it's friends, family, fellow individuals with diabetes, or healthcare providers, the support you receive plays a vital role in your emotional well-being and diabetes management. The chapters have guided you in communicating about your diabetes, building a support network, and engaging with peers who share similar experiences. Your support system is not just a source of encouragement but a community that understands the nuances of living with diabetes.

Looking Ahead with Optimism

As you stand at the conclusion of this book, it's important to look ahead with optimism. Your journey with diabetes is not defined by limitations but by the possibilities of growth, resilience, and a fulfilling life. The knowledge you've acquired, the strategies you've implemented, and the support you've cultivated are tools that empower you to face the future with confidence.

Moving Forward:

1. **Continuous Learning:** The field of diabetes management is dynamic, with ongoing research and advancements. Stay curious and engaged in continuous learning. Explore new developments, attend workshops, and remain informed about emerging technologies and strategies that can enhance your diabetes management.

2. **Regular Health Check-ups:** Regular health check-ups are not just a part of your past; they are integral to your future. These appointments provide opportunities for monitoring your diabetes, addressing concerns, and adjusting your care plan as needed. Commit to attending regular check-ups to stay proactive in managing your health.

3. **Adapting and Growing:** Your journey with diabetes is a journey of adaptation and growth. Be open to adapting

your strategies, learning from experiences, and discovering new approaches that align with your evolving needs. Every challenge is an opportunity for growth, and your ability to adapt is a testament to your resilience.

4. **Celebrating Milestones:** Continue celebrating milestones, both big and small. Your journey is a series of accomplishments, and each achievement is a step toward a more fulfilling life with diabetes. Whether it's reaching a health goal, mastering a new aspect of diabetes management, or cultivating a positive mindset, take the time to acknowledge and celebrate these victories.

5. **Sharing Your Story:** Your experiences and insights are valuable not only to your journey but also to others facing similar challenges. Consider sharing your story with the diabetes community. Whether it's through online platforms, support groups, or community events, your journey can inspire and offer hope to others.

Final Words of Encouragement

In concluding this book, remember that living well with diabetes is not a destination but a continuous journey. It's a journey that intertwines with your everyday life, shaping your experiences, relationships, and personal growth. You are not defined by your diabetes; rather, you define how diabetes fits into your life.

As you navigate the path ahead, carry with you the knowledge gained, the resilience cultivated, and the support system nurtured. Embrace the growth opportunities, celebrate your victories, and approach each day with a spirit of curiosity and optimism. Your journey is uniquely yours, and every step forward is a testament to your strength, courage, and capacity to live a fulfilling life with diabetes.

In the grand tapestry of life, diabetes is but one thread. Your story, with its challenges and triumphs, is woven with threads of resilience, hope, and the power to embrace a new life with diabetes. May your journey be filled with self-discovery, moments of joy, and the unwavering belief in your ability to thrive, not despite diabetes but because of the strength it inspires within you.

As you close this chapter and step into the next phase of your journey, remember that you are not alone. The diabetes community is vast and supportive, and your healthcare team is a reliable ally. Your journey is a testament to your courage and determination. With the knowledge, strategies, and support gained, you are well-equipped to not only manage diabetes but to thrive and lead a life that is rich, meaningful, and uniquely yours.

Here's to embracing your new life with diabetes—a life filled with possibilities, resilience, and the power to thrive.

APPENDIX

Resources, Recipes, and Additional Information

Congratulations on reaching the end of "Living Well With Diabetes for the Newly Diagnosed." In this appendix, you'll find a curated collection of valuable resources, delicious recipes, and additional information to support your journey with diabetes. These resources are designed to complement the information provided in the main chapters, offering practical tools and inspiration for your ongoing diabetes management.

1. Diabetes Resources:

Websites:

- American Diabetes Association: A comprehensive resource providing information on diabetes management, lifestyle, and support.

- JDRF (formerly Juvenile Diabetes Research Foundation): Focuses on type 1 diabetes research, advocacy, and community support.

- Diabetes Forecast: A publication of the American Diabetes Association offering articles, recipes, and tips for living well with diabetes.

- CDC Diabetes: The Centers for Disease Control and Prevention's diabetes resource with information on prevention, management, and statistics.

- Diabetes Daily: An online community providing forums, articles, and resources for people living with diabetes.

Mobile Apps:

- <u>MyFitnessPal</u>: A popular app for tracking nutrition and exercise, helping with meal planning, and maintaining a healthy lifestyle.

- <u>Blood Sugar Tracker by MyNetDiary</u>: A user-friendly app for tracking blood sugar levels, meals, and physical activity.

- <u>Fooducate</u>: Scan barcodes to get personalized nutrition information and healthy food recommendations.

- <u>Diabetes:M</u>: A comprehensive app for tracking blood glucose, medications, meals, and physical activity.

- <u>Carb Manager</u>: A useful app for managing carbohydrate intake, tracking meals, and supporting low-carb lifestyles.

2. Delicious Diabetes-Friendly Recipes:

Breakfast:

- **Greek Yogurt Parfait:**
    - Ingredients:
        - 1 cup Greek yogurt (unsweetened)
        - 1/2 cup berries (strawberries, blueberries, or raspberries)
        - 1 tablespoon chopped nuts (almonds or walnuts)
        - 1 teaspoon honey (optional)

- Instructions:
    - In a glass or bowl, layer Greek yogurt with berries.
    - Top with chopped nuts.
    - Drizzle with honey if desired.

Lunch:

- **Grilled Chicken Salad:**
  - Ingredients:
    - 4 oz grilled chicken breast, sliced
    - 2 cups mixed salad greens
    - 1/2 cup cherry tomatoes, halved
    - 1/4 cucumber, sliced
    - 1 tablespoon olive oil and balsamic vinegar dressing
  - Instructions:
    - Arrange salad greens on a plate.
    - Top with grilled chicken, cherry tomatoes, and cucumber.
    - Drizzle with olive oil and balsamic vinegar dressing.

Dinner:

- **Baked Salmon with Lemon and Herbs:**
  - Ingredients:

- 6 oz salmon fillet

- 1 tablespoon olive oil

- 1 lemon, sliced

- 1 teaspoon dried herbs (rosemary, thyme, or dill)

- Salt and pepper to taste

- Instructions:

  - Preheat oven to 375°F (190°C).

  - Place salmon on a baking sheet.

  - Drizzle with olive oil and season with salt, pepper, and dried herbs.

  - Arrange lemon slices on top.

  - Bake for 15-20 minutes or until salmon is cooked through.

Snack:

- **Vegetable Sticks with Hummus:**

  - Ingredients:

    - 1 cup assorted vegetable sticks (carrots, celery, bell peppers)

    - 2 tablespoons hummus

  - Instructions:

    - Cut vegetables into sticks.

- Serve with hummus for a delicious and nutritious snack.

3. Additional Information:

Books:

- "Think Like a Pancreas" by Gary Scheiner: A guide to managing diabetes with practical advice on insulin, nutrition, and lifestyle.

- "The Diabetes Code" by Dr. Jason Fung: Explores the role of intermittent fasting in managing and preventing type 2 diabetes.

- "Bright Spots & Landmines" by Adam Brown: A personal guide to diabetes management, focusing on practical tips for better living.

Podcasts:

- The Diabetes Connection: Hosted by Stacey Simms, this podcast covers a wide range of topics related to diabetes management, research, and personal stories.

- Diabetes Daily Grind: Real-life stories and conversations about the daily challenges and triumphs of living with diabetes.

- The Juicebox Podcast: Hosted by Scott Benner, this podcast covers various aspects of living with type 1 diabetes, featuring interviews and insights.

Online Communities:

- TuDiabetes: An online community where individuals with diabetes can connect, share experiences, and seek support.

- <u>Beyond Type 1</u>: A platform offering resources, community support, and advocacy for those living with diabetes.

- Diabetes Daily Forum: A community forum where people with diabetes can discuss various topics, share tips, and seek advice.

Educational Videos:

- Diabetes: Understanding the Basics: A comprehensive video explaining the basics of diabetes, its types, and management.

- Blood Sugar and Insulin: An informative video on how blood sugar and insulin work in the body.

- Cooking for Diabetes: A cooking show featuring diabetes-friendly recipes and nutrition tips.

Feel free to explore these resources, try out the recipes, and use the information to enhance your diabetes management journey. Remember, knowledge, community support, and a positive mindset are powerful tools for living well with diabetes. If you have any questions or seek further guidance, don't hesitate to reach out to your healthcare team or fellow individuals in the diabetes community. Wishing you a vibrant and fulfilling life on your journey with diabetes!

GLOSSARY

Key Terms and Definitions for Diabetes Management

Understanding the terminology associated with diabetes management is crucial for navigating your journey effectively. This glossary provides key terms and definitions to help you grasp the language of diabetes care.

1. A1c (HbA1c):

- A blood test that measures the average blood glucose levels over the past 2-3 months. It is expressed as a percentage and is a key indicator of long-term blood sugar control.

2. Basal Insulin:

- A type of insulin that provides a steady release of insulin throughout the day and night, helping to control fasting and between-meal blood glucose levels.

3. Bolus Insulin:

- A type of insulin taken at mealtime to manage the increase in blood glucose that occurs after eating. It is based on the amount of carbohydrates in the meal.

4. Carbohydrate Counting:

- A method of meal planning that involves tracking the amount of carbohydrates in food to help determine the appropriate insulin dose for managing blood sugar levels.

5. Continuous Glucose Monitoring (CGM):

- A system that continuously measures glucose levels throughout the day and night. It provides real-time data and trends, helping individuals make informed decisions about their diabetes management.

6. Dawn Phenomenon:

- The natural rise in blood sugar levels that occurs in the early morning hours, often due to hormonal changes. It can require adjustments to insulin doses.

7. Diabetic Ketoacidosis (DKA):

- A severe and potentially life-threatening complication of diabetes, usually associated with high blood sugar levels. It is characterized by the presence of ketones in the blood.

8. Gestational Diabetes:

- Diabetes that develops during pregnancy. It increases the risk of complications for both the mother and baby and requires careful management.

9. Glucagon:

- A hormone produced by the pancreas that raises blood sugar levels. It is often used as an emergency treatment for severe hypoglycemia.

10. Insulin Resistance:

- A condition where the body's cells do not respond effectively to insulin, leading to higher blood sugar levels. It is common in type 2 diabetes.

11. Ketones:

- Chemicals produced when the body breaks down fat for energy. High levels of ketones can occur in conditions like diabetic ketoacidosis.

12. LADA (Latent Autoimmune Diabetes in Adults):

- A form of autoimmune diabetes that resembles type 1 diabetes but typically develops in adults. It progresses more slowly than typical type 1 diabetes.

13. Microvascular Complications:

- Diabetes-related complications that affect small blood vessels, including retinopathy (eye damage), nephropathy (kidney damage), and neuropathy (nerve damage).

14. Macrovascular Complications:

- Diabetes-related complications that affect large blood vessels, increasing the risk of heart disease, stroke, and peripheral vascular disease.

15. Oral Glucose Tolerance Test (OGTT):

- A diagnostic test that measures how the body responds to a glucose load. It is often used to diagnose gestational diabetes and can provide insights into insulin sensitivity.

16. Pancreas:

- An organ that produces insulin and other hormones. In diabetes, the pancreas may not produce enough insulin or the body may not use it effectively.

17. Polyphagia, Polydipsia, Polyuria:

- Symptoms of diabetes. Polyphagia refers to increased hunger, polydipsia to increased thirst, and polyuria to increased urination.

18. Type 1 Diabetes:

- An autoimmune condition where the immune system attacks and destroys the insulin-producing beta cells in the pancreas. It requires lifelong insulin therapy.

19. Type 2 Diabetes:

- A condition characterized by insulin resistance and inadequate insulin production. It is often managed with lifestyle changes, oral medications, and, in some cases, insulin.

20. Hypoglycemia:

- A condition characterized by low blood sugar levels, often resulting in symptoms such as shakiness, confusion, and sweating. It is usually treated with fast-acting carbohydrates.

This glossary provides a foundation for understanding key terms related to diabetes management. Keep in mind that effective communication with your healthcare team is essential for personalized care. If you encounter terms not covered here or have specific questions, don't hesitate to seek clarification from your healthcare provider.